SUCCESSFUL ACADEMIC WRITING

Also Available

*Qualitative Inquiry
in Clinical and Educational Settings*
Danica G. Hays and Anneliese Singh

SUCCESSFUL ACADEMIC WRITING

A Complete Guide for Social and Behavioral Scientists

Anneliese A. Singh
Lauren Lukkarila

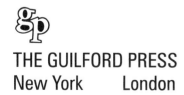

THE GUILFORD PRESS
New York   London

*For all of our past, current, and future students and mentors
with whom we have shared the academic writing road*

*For our mothers—Diane Singh and Peggy Phillips—
who taught us a love of reading
and, therefore, a love of writing*

And for Malakai, Id, and Bibi, with boundless love

Copyright © 2017 The Guilford Press
A Division of Guilford Publications, Inc.
370 Seventh Avenue, Suite 1200, New York, NY 10001
www.guilford.com

Printed in the United States of America

This book is printed on acid-free paper.

Last digit is print number: 9   8   7   6   5   4   3   2

Library of Congress Cataloging-in-Publication Data

Names: Singh, Anneliese A., author.
Title: Successful academic writing : a complete guide for social and
    behavioral scientists / Anneliese A. Singh, Lauren Lukkarila.
Description: New York : The Guilford Press, 2017. | Includes bibliographical
    references and index.
Identifiers: LCCN 2016049552| ISBN 9781462529391 (paperback) | ISBN
    9781462529407 (hardcover)
Subjects: LCSH: Academic writing. | Social science literature. | BISAC:
    LANGUAGE ARTS & DISCIPLINES / Composition & Creative Writing. | REFERENCE
    / Writing Skills. | MEDICAL / Education & Training. | SOCIAL SCIENCE /
    Research. | PSYCHOLOGY / Research & Methodology. | EDUCATION / Research.
Classification: LCC P301.5.A27 S56 2017 | DDC 808.02/3—dc23
LC record available at *https://lccn.loc.gov/2016049552*

Preface

Our collaboration on this book grew from many mutual conversations about writing. Anneliese works with counseling and psychology graduate students in the United States, and Lauren works with English language learners in higher education from around the world. When we would talk about our shared experiences of teaching about writing, we had lively discussions and debates and swapped pedagogical strategies and encouragement for this work. As these conversations continued—often while burning the midnight oil—we began to realize we had a book on our hands. We were so passionate about writing, specifically about supporting student writing, that we decided that, yep, we wanted to write this book.

A large part of our excitement has been grounded in how we see the students we work with progress from talking about academic writing as though it is something to be avoided at all costs to developing confidence in their own voices as academic writers. We also have talked endlessly about how many of our students enter our classes woefully unprepared for academic writing owing to inadequate support and resources during their earlier education. We also saw students struggle to believe that they could write.

As we became more and more curious about why this lack of preparation for and confidence about academic writing existed for most students, we had many "aha!" moments. We remembered the teachers who encouraged us to write and told us we were good writers. We also remembered our parents, who took us to libraries and cultivated a love of reading—and, therefore, a love of writing. We were not just lucky in these regards; we see these experiences and resources as aspects of privilege that many students whom we work with did not have before they entered our classrooms or any graduate setting. We noted that we could use this privilege to convey to our current students that they *can* learn academic writing, and even become strong academic writers along the way.

So, in writing this book, we have been guided by our late-night conversations about academic writing, our love of teaching, and our appreciation for our past, current, and future students who open themselves to learning and growing as academic writers. Our aim has been to dispel myths about academic writing and to unlock the "secrets" that seem to exist about it. No one told us about the secrets of academic writing, either, and we "figured it out," just like most people. We want our book to be a part of the solution, so that students do not have to wonder what they missed or whether they are prepared for good academic writing. This book is all about spelling out those secrets and unspoken rules and breaking apart the nitty-gritty steps of academic writing.

To do this, we divided this book into three sections. In Unit I, "Becoming an Academic Writer," Chapter 1, *What Is Academic Writing?,* talks about what academic writing is and is *not.* Chapter 2, *Preparing for Writing Success in Your Discipline,* is geared toward getting you ready to learn the specific academic practices within your discipline or community of practice (CoP). Chapter 3, *Developing Your Own Writing Identity,* helps bring you back to your own writing identity and develop your voice as a writer.

In Unit II, "Developing Academic Writing Skills," we venture into the specific skills that will move your writing forward, making you a stronger and leaner writer. Chapter 4, *Understanding Academic Writer–Reader Roles and Writing Structures,* and Chapter 5, *The Use of Tone and Style in Your Academic Writing,* will help you understand how those within your CoP use their writing to innovate ideas and push the field forward. In these two companion chapters, we talk about how the issues of coherence, writer–reader rules, and audience awareness, as well as rational tone and cohesive style, play into your academic writing. In Chapter 6, *Coaching Yourself to Completion,* we discuss strategies for getting your writing started, moving, and completed, and also talk about specific coaching tips that help you enjoy your writing.

By the time we get to Unit III, "Specific Types of Academic Writing," you will have unlocked a good number of secrets about academic writing and have a solid toolkit of skills and strategies under your belt. Thus it is time to delve into the specific types of academic writing. So in Chapter 7, *Grounding Your Voice in the Literature,* we discuss how to write standalone literature reviews. In Chapter 8, *The Writing Formula for Empirical Academic Writing,* we describe how to write standard sections of empirical (e.g., qualitative, quantitative, mixed-methods) articles as an academic writer. We conclude this unit and the text with Chapter 9, *Publish, Don't Perish,* discussing how you might jump into the publishing world with the support of and trust in what you already know about academic writing.

Throughout this book, we include numerous text boxes, practices, tables, and figures to bring to life the strategies of academic writing. We encourage you to read chapter content and then really engage in these focused learning opportunities. There is also an Appendix—an answer key for some of the practices in which we ask you to identify important academic writing moves within author texts. We have intentionally embedded peer-reviewed journal article exemplars of academic writing so you can see how the strategies we are talking about are explicitly used by published authors. We also begin each chapter with an *awareness focus,* related to the chapter content, and then an *action focus.* These foci are intended to keep you thinking about the overall why-is-this-important points within each chapter. At the end of each chapter, we summarize awareness and action reminders so you have a bit of a snapshot of the chapters as well. Our writing style is honest and straightforward and aims to lead you step by step in becoming a stronger academic writer than you ever might have imagined. You can see that practicality, accessibility, and usefulness were our guideposts in compiling this book. We hope you enjoy reading it as much as we enjoyed dreaming it up and bringing it to fruition.

A brief note about pronouns: With the exception of specific examples, we will be alternating between masculine and feminine pronouns throughout the book to avoid awkward sentences.

Acknowledgments

We would like to express great appreciation to the people who supported our book idea from inception to publication. To C. Deborah Laughton at The Guilford Press, we have appreciated your guidance, clear vision, good humor, and unwavering support as we have developed this text. It is rare to work with a publisher who expresses such care and concern not only for the topic of the book, but for us as authors. We look forward to many more coffee dates with you in the future! We would also like to express our gratitude to the phenomenal reviewers for our text, who provided thoughtful commentary and challenged us to address common concerns and gaps in academic writing: Susan P. Robbins (Graduate College of Social Work, University of Houston); Peggy Meszaros (Department of Human Development, Virginia Tech); Vanessa P. Dennen (College of Education, Florida State University; Editor-in-Chief, *The Internet and Higher Education*); Ann Marie Ryan (Department of Psychology, Michigan State University); and Patricia Goodson (Health and Kinesiology, Texas A&M University). Our book is much stronger and will be more helpful to our readers as a result of the time you spent providing your reviews. Many thanks as well to Paul Gordon, who designed a wonderful cover that captures the many coffee tables and coffee houses where we actually wrote this text! To Oliver Sharpe, who provided stellar interior design and typesetting for the book, we very much appreciated your fine eye for detail. For her patience and steadfast communication, we thank Jeannie Tang for serving as our main contact overseeing the publication of our book and keeping us on track.

Contents

UNIT I
BECOMING AN ACADEMIC WRITER

CHAPTER 1

What Is Academic Writing?

Academic writing in the behavioral and social sciences is a way of writing that is *distinctly different* from other forms of writing. On the surface, it may appear to have similarities with other types of writing, but the more you learn about it, the more you realize that just about every aspect of academic writing, from purpose to tone, from structure to style, and from audience to word choice, is different. Quite literally, academic writing is more than just another way to write; it is a different culture with its own language.

So, how do you learn academic writing? This is the question that guides this book. We believe that the basic equation for any kind of learning is awareness + action = growth. In your case, this means we believe you will experience positive development as an academic writer if you do the following:

1. Develop *awareness* of academic writing—that is, develop factual knowledge about it as a culture and a language.

2. Take *action* to increase your membership in the academic writing culture and your fluency in academic writing language—that is, consciously and diligently do things that improve your skills and strategies for accomplishing academic writing at a level that is satisfactory for accomplishing your goals.

Accordingly, in this book, our goal is to provide you with a balance of *awareness* (knowledge) and *action* (skill/strategy development steps) in an effort to facilitate growth in your academic writing. Our belief is that expertise in anything—but especially something as specific as academic writing—is primarily a result of extensive practice. As Malcolm Gladwell engagingly illustrates in *Outliers: The Story of Success* (2008), it is 10,000 hours of practice, rather than just inherent ability, that to some extent distinguishes a "phenom" from others in a field. Of course, we do not expect you to make 10,000 hours of practice in academic writing your goal. We just want to emphasize that all time spent *understanding and practicing* academic writing will result in increasing your academic writing expertise.

In this first chapter, our **awareness focus** is helping you to gain an understanding of what academic writing *is*—and what academic writing is *not*. Our **action focus** includes ideas for steps you can take to consciously develop your ability to see written texts through the eyes of an academic writer. Let's begin by exploring what academic writing *is* and is *not* in more detail.

DEFINING ACADEMIC WRITING

Academic writing is more than just another way to write; it is literally a different culture with its own language. In fact, academic writing is more than just one different culture. It is simultaneously one culture and many cultures, which can obviously create confusion for those trying to join the culture(s) and learn the language(s). Academic writing is one culture in the sense that most experienced, successful academic writers (from the same country) would likely agree on several of the general qualities of academic writing. However, academic writing is also many cultures because those same experienced, successful academic writers would also likely look at the same academically written text and provide very different comments and suggestions for revisions based on what is considered the norm in their specific discipline. Thus, even people like your professors, who operate very successfully within the culture and language of academic writing, may have a difficult time of breaking down what is and what is not academic writing in explicit terms, because it is not one thing. It is many things, and they did not *learn* it—they *absorbed* it. Right now, if you were to schedule a meeting with your favorite professor and ask her to define what academic writing is, you might get some vague answers like the following:

- "It is what we use in writing journal articles."
- "You know academic writing when you see it."
- "You know what is *not* academic writing when you see it."
- "Academic writing is formal, neutral language."

Of course, the confusing thing about these types of responses is that they do not really answer your question. You still do not know what academic writing is, and as far as you can tell at this point, neither does your professor. So, how are you supposed to figure out how to do academic writing when you do not know what it is? Perhaps you should ask your professor another question, such as, "How did you learn academic writing?" This time, you may get more concrete responses:

- "I had to learn academic writing on my own."
- "I learned academic writing when I was working on my dissertation."
- "Academic writing was really varied according to my professors. I picked up a little something from each professor I worked with in graduate school."
- "I am still learning what academic writing is—it seems to change according to journal, colleague, and discipline!"

Although these answers may also seem unhelpful, you can begin to understand that professors have difficulty defining what academic writing is because they likely experienced very little direct instruction in developing themselves as academic writers. Like you, they were expected to produce academic writing that met some mysterious standard defined by their professors, and somehow (they may not know how) they managed to achieve that standard.

The journey to becoming an academic writer is unique and highly individualized for everyone, and inevitably involves some strategic planning, some trial and error, and lots of perseverance. Thus the first major awareness that can help move you forward in your own process of becoming an academic writer is to understand that you are in charge of this journey. It will ultimately be up to you to direct your own process of becoming an academic writer and to figure out what works for you. The key action that can help you to take charge of your journey is to be curious. Curiosity will lead you not only to notice things you need to notice in your journey to becoming an academic writer, but also to seek explanations, resources, and assistance as you manage your journey. For example, curiosity will help you to develop the ability to see written texts as experienced academic writers see them, and this is a crucial step in your process of becoming an academic writer.

ACADEMIC WRITING VERSUS OTHER TYPES OF WRITING

Is a magazine article academic writing? Is a newspaper editorial academic writing? Is an advertising brochure academic writing? What about a blog post? Text message? Tweet? Is an office memo academic writing? A recipe . . . e-mail . . . message taped to your door . . . or a to-do list? We think you get our point. Chances are you said "No" to all of the above. If so, you are generally correct. Each of those types of writing is common—so common you may read and/or write them every day—but none of them are academic writing.

At the same time, academic writing is not a single type of text. The categorization of something as academic writing generally means that the something in question shares a specific combination of features that are considered representative of the term *academic*. In what might be considered "good" academic writing, these features include but are not limited to the following:

- *Audience awareness.* The intended or imagined audience or reader for the text is clearly envisioned as having some shared knowledge about the content.

- *Argumentative purpose.* The purpose of the text is to argue an overall position or point of view about a topic that is in some way new or unique by demonstrating knowledge about the topic and ability to use that knowledge.

- *Problematizating approach.* The overall position or point of view on a topic typically presents previous positions or points of view as problematic in some way, even when those previous positions or points of view may have been long accepted as common knowledge. The goal of such an approach is generally to create a rationale for considering the topic from new or alternative points of view.

- *Rational tone.* The writer of the text assumes the reader will be either appeased or persuaded by the obvious and carefully explained logic of the argument.

- *Relevant content.* The text includes only academically credible information that is relevant to supporting and forwarding the writer's argument or discrediting information that does not support the writer's argument.

- *Coherent structure.* Regardless of the relative length of the text, it must follow a precise organizational plan on a macro-level, as in the case of the organization of an academic research article, and on a meso-level, as in the case of a single paragraph of an academic research article. The academic coherence is reflected in the way ideas are introduced and broken down for further discussion. In academic writing, ideas are introduced categorically, from general categories to more specific categories to even more specific instances of those categories.

- *Cohesive style.* The writer assumes more or less complete responsibility for the reader's understanding of his ideas and uses linguistic devices such as repetition of key words, parallel structure, transition words or expressions, and a sophisticated variety of synonyms or metaphors to create writing that tightly connects ideas, leaving little room for misinterpretations. This style includes significant attention to establishing definitions and clarifying relationships between ideas to ensure that the reader sees things in the manner intended by the writer.

- *Complex, but not ornate, grammar and vocabulary.* The writer utilizes different sentence types, alternates between active and passive voice, and generally composes with a wide range of precise and sometimes technical vocabulary. However, the complexity of the grammar and vocabulary does not diminish the clarity of the argument, even for those who may not be necessarily trained in that particular content area.

Successful use of the aforementioned features generally produces "good" academic writing. Understanding how experienced writers in your field specifically accomplish these features and acquiring the ability to do the same helps you develop a writing "voice" that is more credible in your field. See Box 1.1 for a summary list of criteria that make your writing credible in the academic world of behavioral and social sciences. These are components of academic writing that professors, journal editors, and reviewers, among others, are typically expecting in your writing.

Notice that, if you were to apply these criteria to other forms of writing, the individual criterion might be fulfilled, but it would not appear in the same way it does in academic writing. For example, audience awareness is a criterion for many forms of writing, including tweeting. If you want people to read your writing with interest, you have to project an imagined audience through the content and style of your writing. If your Twitter followers are

---

BOX 1.1. Criteria for Credible Academic Writing in Behavioral and Social Sciences

- Audience = Academic
- Purpose = Argumentation
- Approach = Problematizing
- Tone = Rational
- Content = Academically credible
- Structure = Highly organized according to logical principles of argumentation
- Style = Highly cohesive to clearly establish connections between ideas
- Language = Clear prose that demonstrates sophisticated and precise knowledge of grammar, vocabulary, and mechanics

eighth-grade boys who love video games and hip-hop, tweeting a satirical response to a political event probably would not maintain or grow your readership. If you tweet, you must appeal to your audience, whoever they happen to be. Similarly, if you write academically, you must appeal to an academic audience, and you must understand what that audience expects.

You can help yourself in this area by taking some simple actions. You already know lots of things about writing that can be useful to you in figuring out the differences between academic writing and other forms of writing. The information is already there for you in your brain and your past experience. The following is a simple pattern of questions you can use to access what you already know so your awareness of what academic writing *is* and *is not* will grow:

1. What kind of writing text is this—how would you categorize it? Is it a news article, a text message, a blog, a personal e-mail, etc.?
2. Who is the likely imagined or intended audience/reader for this text?
3. What is the purpose of this text? Why did the writer write it? What impact or effect does the writer want it to have on the reader?
4. How did the writer approach the topic of this text? What strategy was used to provide a basic rationale for writing about this topic?
5. What type of information is included in this text? Is it all closely related to one central idea, or does the information introduce many different ideas?
6. What is the tone of this text? What is the attitude of the writer toward the reader?
7. What is the structure or organization of ideas in this text? Does it appear to have some kind of formal structure, is it stream of consciousness, or is it something in between?
8. What is the style of expression used in this text? Are the ideas tightly connected and clearly explained in relation to each other? Are the ideas presented somewhat sequentially but not necessarily explained?
9. What kind of grammar and vocabulary are used in this text? Are the sentences simple or complex? Is the vocabulary sophisticated, requiring a high level of literacy, or is it more conversational?
10. Based on your answers to numbers 1–9, how does this text you are currently evaluating compare to academic writing?

If you regularly practice analyzing any written text you encounter with these questions, before long you will have a very clear idea of how all forms of writing compare to one another. You will also develop a more nuanced understanding of how the seemingly small differences between texts can make such a huge difference when it comes to producing written texts that readers judge as fitting their intended categories. You will begin to see texts through the eyes of an academic writer. Try your hand at analyzing differences between texts by answering the questions in Practice Exercise 1.1. You can check your answers in the Appendix.

PRACTICE EXERCISE 1.1. Identifying Text Type

TEXT 1

Worried about the past? Stressed out about the future? How do you feel right now? Mindfulness is a practice you can use to move into the **NOW moment**, and that move can make you happier and calmer.

When your mind is busy reliving the past and thinking about what you could have or should have done, you lose energy. The past is a movie you've already seen—seeing it again won't change the outcome! When your mind is busy inventing an unknown future and stressing about what might go wrong, you lose energy. The future is a game that hasn't started yet—you can't play it before it begins! So, stop, breathe in, look around, and notice: **What are you doing right now? How do you feel right now? What do you see, hear, taste, and smell right now?**

Questions for Text 1

1. What kind of writing text is Text 1—how would you categorize it? Is it a news article, a blog, a personal e-mail, a Web page, a brochure, an abstract for a research article, a book review, part of a literature review, part of a Method section, or part of a Discussion section?
2. Who is the likely imagined or intended audience/reader for this text?
3. What is the purpose of this text? Why did the author write it? What impact or effect does the author want it to have on the reader?
4. How did the author approach the topic of this text? What strategy was used to provide a basic rationale for writing about this topic?
5. What type of information is included in this text? Is it all closely related to one central idea, or does the information introduce many different ideas?
6. What is the tone of this text? What is the attitude of the author toward the reader?
7. What is the structure or organization of ideas in this text? Does it appear to have some kind of formal structure, is it stream of consciousness, or is it something in between?
8. What is the style of expression used in this text? Are the ideas tightly

connected and clearly explained in relation to each other? Are the ideas presented somewhat sequentially but not necessarily explained?

9. What kind of grammar and vocabulary are used in this text? Are the sentences simple or complex? Is the vocabulary sophisticated, requiring a high level of literacy, or is it more conversational?

10. Based on your answers to numbers 1–9, how does this text that you are currently evaluating compare to academic writing?

TEXT 2
(Gould, Dariotis, Mendelson, & Greenberg, 2012, p. 968)

Mindfulness practices that utilize yoga and other contemplative techniques are a promising approach for enhancing key aspects of self-regulation (e.g., Chiesa & Serretti, 2009; Greenberg & Harris, 2011; Lutz et al., 2009; Tang et al., 2009). Derived from Eastern contemplative traditions, *mindfulness* involves attending to the present moment in a sustained and receptive fashion (Brown & Ryan, 2003). Yoga, a specific form of mindfulness, involves maintaining focused attention on one's breath and body while performing movements that improve strength and flexibility. Indeed, the Sanskrit root of "yoga" means "to yoke, to join, and to direct and concentrate one's attention" (Collins, 1998, p. 564). Yoga and other meditative techniques have been shown to increase attention and self-regulation and reduce stress and improve functioning in adults (Arias, Steinberg, Banga, & Trestment, 2006; Kirkwood et al., 2005; Ospina et al., 2007; Pilkington, Kirkwood, Rampes, & Richardson, 2005; Shapiro, Brown, & Biegel, 2007).

Questions for Text 2

1. What kind of writing text is Text 2—how would you categorize it? Is it a news article, a blog, a personal e-mail, a Web page, a brochure, an abstract for a research article, a book review, part of a literature review, part of a Method section, or part of a Discussion section?

2. Who is the likely imagined or intended audience/reader for this text?

3. What is the purpose of this text? Why did the author write it? What impact or effect does the author want it to have on the reader?

4. How did the author approach the topic of this text? What strategy was used to provide a basic rationale for writing about this topic?

5. What type of information is included in this text? Is it all closely related to one central idea, or does the information introduce many different ideas?

6. What is the tone of this text? What is the attitude of the author toward the reader?

7. What is the structure or organization of ideas in this text? Does it appear to have some kind of formal structure, is it stream of consciousness, or is it something in between?

8. What is the style of expression used in this text? Are the ideas tightly connected and clearly explained in relation to each other? Are the ideas presented somewhat sequentially but not necessarily explained?

9. What kind of grammar and vocabulary are used in this text? Are the sentences simple or complex? Is the vocabulary sophisticated, requiring a high level of literacy, or is it more conversational?

10. Based on your answers to numbers 1–9, how does this text that you are currently evaluating compare to academic writing?

EVERYDAY CONVERSATIONAL LANGUAGE VERSUS ACADEMIC WRITING LANGUAGE

Although language style is a consideration that we have briefly touched on in discussing differences between academic and nonacademic texts, the topic of language style merits a little more attention because it is such a distinguishing characteristic of academic writing and because it is also such a common mistake for new academic writers. In your—hopefully daily—evaluation of different written texts, you have probably noticed that texts can discuss the exact same ideas using many different words and styles of expression. Some written texts, such as text messages, tweets, and personal e-mails, use a conversational style of language that is very similar if not identical to speaking language. Some, such as news articles and advertisements, use a journalistic or media style of language that is very emotional and intensifying but not terribly sophisticated. Others, such as memos, recipes, and to-do lists, prefer a directive style of language that is instructional. Some, such as academic research articles, use a language we simply refer to as academic writing language. Academic writing language is something like Latin in the sense that it is a language people learn to read and write, but it is not actually a language they speak.

As new graduate students, it is particularly important that you become aware of the differences between what may be considered acceptable language for talking about concepts during class discussions and what is acceptable language for writing about concepts in written assignments. The language of class discussions is often very conversational, and this can be misleading if you mistake the way something is discussed in class for the way you should discuss it in writing. Learning the language of academic writing, particularly the language of academic writing in your discipline, is essential to your development as an academic writer.

As we mentioned earlier, developing your ability to see written texts as experienced academic writers do is a fundamental building block for developing your own academic writing voice. One of the basic rules for learning any language—academic or otherwise—is that input informs output, or what you can do with language (output) is a reflection of what language you have absorbed (input). Thus, the more you are exposed to academic writing language in what you read, the more likely it is that this language will become one of your own languages. However, simple exposure is not enough and will not give you the results you want quickly enough. Your exposure to academic writing language needs to be intentional and conscious. You cannot just wait for academic writing language to gradually seep into your awareness; you have to actively pursue the input you need. To increase your intentional and conscious exposure to the academic writing language of your discipline, we suggest that graduate students take the following actions:

- Immerse yourself in academic writing language by truly and carefully reading all of the assignments your professors give. Treat every reading assignment as another opportunity to "learn the lingo" of your discipline.

- Take notes, write summaries, give oral summaries, and even engage in academic discussions using the same kind of language that was used in the academic texts you read to practice the academic writing language you are learning. It might seem like extra work or you may even feel pretentious, but in the long run, you are preparing yourself for academic writing.

- Keep a list of words or phrases or even sentences that seem to be frequently used in your discipline. Every field has its buzzwords, shorthand, and special ways of communicating information to other members of the field. Each time your professors ask you to read multiple articles on the same topic, you are being given the opportunity to notice the similar language all of the writers used to discuss the same topic. If you have something like Adobe Acrobat, you can often cut and paste words or sentences into a separate document, so keeping a list is not all that hard.

DIFFERENT TYPES OF ACADEMIC READING AND WRITING

Even though we have encouraged you to see academic writing as different from other types of writing, and we still want you to do that, we also want to acknowledge that not all academic writing is the same, despite the fact that it is all academic. Graduate syllabi may include a variety of texts to read, such as textbooks, academic research articles, case studies, monographs, and chapters from edited books, as well as nonfiction and fiction books, editorials, blogs, and Web pages, among others. Some of these texts are considered "academic," and some of them are not. However, when they are read within an academic context such as a graduate course, you can be sure that you are expected to read, discuss, and use them in academic ways.

Although the designation of academic versus nonacademic text could be and has been debated, for our purposes, we propose that academic texts are those texts you read that you probably would not choose to read except in the pursuit of building an academic knowledge base. For example, textbooks, case studies, academic research articles of all kinds, monographs, chapters from edited books, theses, and dissertations are probably not the kind of reading you would randomly select for your personal reading list. Even though their topics might interest you personally, the academic style of expression used in these types of texts might be off-putting for casual reading.

Most of us are intimately familiar with the textbook as an academic text, having used them for probably every course of our student lives. We have probably also seen case studies before, at least in miniature versions, because they are frequently included in textbooks. On the other hand, graduate school may be our first "real" introduction to other types of academic texts such as research articles, monographs, chapters from edited books, theses, and dissertations.

The following is a list of what we consider to be academic texts, along with a few important facts about each that we think are important for graduate readers and writers in the behavioral and social sciences to know. It is not an exhaustive list, but includes some of the major types of academic writing you will come across in your studies.

Textbooks

A textbook is a book-length summary of what is considered standard knowledge in a specific topic area. Standard characteristics include the following:

- They are divided into chapters, sections, and subsections.
- They are typically written in an objective or neutral point of view, although there are exceptions.
- They generally contain common knowledge in a given field and/or information summarized from secondary sources.
- They repeat and deepen ideas and constructs related to a topic.
- They include lots of field-specific vocabulary and definitions.
- They are written in a friendly but formal style that is intended to simplify ideas for the reader, who is presumed to know less than the writer.

Case Vignettes

A case vignette is a story-like illustration of a problem or potential problem in a specific field that varies from a few sentences to multiple pages. Standard characteristics include the following:

- They may be hypothetical or based on real-life situations.
- They generally include both relevant and nonrelevant information.
- They may be written in a report style (i.e., here are the facts) or may follow a fiction (i.e., story-like) style.

Research Articles

Scholars publish peer-reviewed articles in academic journals. All fields are represented by multiple journals that publish research in their discipline. Articles are typically anonymous and peer-reviewed by other researchers within a topic area before they are published to ensure the quality and credibility of the research. A mistaken assumption new graduate students may have is that professors are paid for their articles or paid for reviewing other researchers' articles. Publishing research articles and reviewing them is unpaid work that is undertaken by professors because it is part of the standard work requirements for obtaining tenure, promotion, and other rewards (raises, awards, etc.). Academic research articles can be roughly divided into four types:

- Empirical studies (i.e., the researchers conducted some type of study).
- Conceptual articles (i.e., the researchers reviewed and interpreted multiple empirical and conceptual studies done by others).
- Propositional articles (i.e., the researchers are proposing new theories or directions that are creative but logical considering other empirical and conceptual research).
- Response articles (i.e., the researchers are responding, usually critically, to research or an idea that was published by another).

Academic research journals all have prescribed requirements in terms of style. For example, some may require following the *Publication Manual of the American Psychological Association* (APA), some the *MLA* (Modern Language Association) *Handbook*, some the *Chicago Manual of Style,* and so on. Research articles are generally quite formulaic in their structure and are presented in titled sections and subsections. The general formula is as follows:

- Introduce the topic and the research problem that will be addressed in a brief introduction.
- Explain the necessary definitions and background information required to understand the research problem and its significance in the field.
- Explain what you (the researcher) have done to investigate this problem, as well as what you have found as a result of your investigation.

- Discuss the significance and meaning of what you have found in relation to the problem and your field.
- Discuss the limitations of what you did and how that may have affected what you found.
- Return to the research problem, explain how what you found furthers knowledge about this problem, and suggest what still needs to be done.

Other standard characteristics of academic research articles include the following:

- Careful and intentional reference to multiple sources throughout.
- Inclusion of a primary argument, even though much of the text is focused on using support from secondary sources.
- Dense prose (i.e., each sentence carries a lot of information).
- Frequent use of technical, field-specific vocabulary, often without definitions.
- A formal style that is intended to share "important" information with a reader who is presumed to be a colleague or soon-to-be colleague in the field.

Monographs

A monograph is a book-length version of an academic research article. As such, the structure and characteristics of a monograph are quite similar to a research article except that, of course, writers have more pages—so they may include more details or explain more than would be possible in a regular research article.

Chapters in Edited Books

A chapter in an edited book might not have a standard form. A researcher is usually invited to submit a chapter to an edited book when that researcher has done interesting or unique work in the topic area of the book. The editors usually tell the researcher the point of view they wish to put forth in the book, and the researcher writes a chapter that adds to or supports this point of view using her own research as illustration. In some ways, a chapter in an edited book is similar to an academic research article, but the focus is typically a self-summary of a researcher's work or point of view on a topic area.

Theses and Dissertations

Theses and dissertations are student-written academic texts, which may also be read and used by both student and professional academic researchers and/or eventually turned into another academic text, such as those described above. These texts usually contain multiple chapters that include introduction, literature review, methods, results, discussion, and conclusion. Standard characteristics of these texts include the following:

- Careful and intentional reference to multiple sources throughout.
- Inclusion of a primary argument, even though much of the text is focused on using support from secondary sources.
- Significant attention to explanation and definition.
- Noticeable hedging (i.e., suggestive rather than conclusive language).
- A formal style that is intended to demonstrate the writer's ability to both do research and write research for a reader who is presumed to already be an established researcher in the field.

For new graduate students, increasing your awareness of the characteristics that distinguish the different types of academic texts you are asked to read is important because, of course, you may eventually be asked to produce different types of academic texts. In addition, much of the academic writing you are asked to do will require you to find and integrate ideas from different academic sources. In order to do this, you will need to understand what types of academic sources are available to you and how to read them in ways that allow you to effectively use their ideas in your own academic writing. Thus, understanding how these texts you read were put together can improve your reading and writing.

In general, academic writing is highly organized and patterned. Each type of text may have its own pattern, and each unique text may follow that pattern in slightly different ways, but the essential pattern is recognizable. In this case, the pattern we are referring to is the overall organization and structure of a text, or, as we call it, the *macro-level* organization. This is the level of organization that is based on the large parts, such as sections or subsections, that make up the whole text. Just as you need to learn academic writing language, you also need to learn academic writing structure and organization. Specifically, you need to understand how the parts of any longer piece of writing are structured and organized to support the writer's argument. To improve your understanding of how different types of texts are organized and structured in your discipline, we suggest the following actions:

- Actively and consciously identify the macro-level pattern of each text you read. Then compare and categorize the texts you read according to their macro-level patterns.
- Save "good" examples of different types of texts in your own files so that, when you later have to produce these texts yourself, you will have ready models to inspire and guide you.

The first action of identifying and comparing macro-level patterns can be achieved by asking yourself a few questions about each text you read. It is actually beneficial to ask yourself these questions *before* you read a text as a way not only to identify the macro-level pattern but also to improve your own understanding of what you read. These questions can help you figure out the central ideas and have some understanding of the argument presented in the text before you begin:

1. Who is the likely imagined or intended audience/reader for this text? Where in the text is this imagined or intended audience/reader first indicated?

2. What is the question this text seeks to answer? Where is this question first indicated? Why does the writer believe that it is important to answer this question?

3. What types of sections and subsections are included, if any? How do these sections and subsections relate to the question the text seeks to answer? Do these sections and subsections suggest that this is a particular type of text (e.g., empirical research article, monograph, etc.)? Explain.

4. Based on your answers to numbers 1–3, how does this academic text you are currently evaluating compare to other academic texts you have read? Is its macro-level pattern similar to other texts, or is it something totally new to you?

In the case of a research article, you can generally answer these questions simply by skimming through the introduction and scanning the article for the headings and subheadings. In Practice Exercise 1.2, we have provided information on the imagined audience and research questions for two different research articles. We have also provided you with a list of the headings used in each article. Use the information we have provided, along with your own interpretative skills, to figure out how the macro-structure relates to the research questions and what the macro-structure reveals about the type of research article each text is. You can check your answers in the Appendix.

PRACTICE EXERCISE 1.2. Comparing Macro-Level Patterns

Review the information about audience and research questions provided about Text 1. Then review the headings and subheadings used in the text. As you review this information, consider the following questions:

1. How do these headings and subheadings relate to the questions that the text seeks to answer?

2. Do these headings and subheadings suggest that this is a particular

type of text (e.g., empirical research article, monograph, etc.)? Explain.

TEXT 1: AUDIENCE/RESEARCH QUESTIONS

Kim (2014) published an article titled "When Social Class Meets Ethnicity: College-Going Experiences of Chinese and Korean Immigrant Students" in *The Review of Higher Education*. Based on our reading of the introduction of the article (the first three paragraphs), Kim's imagined or intended audience is college admissions officers or college administrators. We inferred this from the use of the following phrases in the first paragraph: "decision to attend college," "college aspirants," "educational aspirations," "college admission processes," "transition to college," "college admission," "college entrance exams," "college education," "college information," and "college application process" (p. 321). For us, the use of so many phrases that focus on college as a next step indicate that the writer expects the audience to be people who are concerned about and responsible for recruiting and/or interacting with students and parents who are looking at college as a next step.

Based on our interpretation of the introduction of the text, the writer seeks to answer the following questions: How do socioeconomic backgrounds affect the involvement of Asian immigrant parents in their children's postsecondary decisions? How do immigrant children negotiate their parents' expectations and involvement in their postsecondary decisions? These questions are indirectly stated in the final paragraph of the introduction. The writer appears to think these questions are important because they have not been as well researched in relation to Asian immigrant parents and children as they have for Asian American parents and children.

Headings/Subheadings

    I. Introduction (not labeled as a heading)

    II. What Accounts for the Educational Outcomes of Asian Immigrants?

    III. Theoretical Perspectives

    IV. Methods

        A. Research Site and Study Participants

    V. Data Collection and Analysis

    VI. Ensuring Data Quality and Reflexivity

    VII. Limitations

    VIII. Findings

        A. College Aspirations: Shaping My Own Future versus Fulfilling My Family's Hopes

        B. Educational Strategies: Co-Ethnic Networks and School Resources

C. Students' Conflict with Utilitarian Parental Expectations for College Majors

D. Choosing the Right College: Financial Affordability Versus Academic Prestige

IX. Discussion and Implication

Review the information about audience and research questions provided about Text 2. Then review the headings and subheadings used in the text. As you review this information, consider the following questions:

1. How do these headings and subheadings relate to the questions that the text seeks to answer?

2. Do these headings and subheadings suggest that this is a particular type of text (empirical research article, monograph, etc.)? Explain.

3. How does the macro-structure of Text 1 compare to the macro-structure of Text 2? Are they the same type of research article? Explain.

TEXT 2: AUDIENCE/RESEARCH QUESTIONS

Hawkins, Manzi, and Ojeda (2014) published an article titled "Lives in the Making: Power, Academia and the Everyday" in *ACME: An International E-Journal for Critical Geographies*. We believe the likely intended audience for this article includes "academic geographers in the making" (or graduate students of geography). This audience is explicitly mentioned and discussed throughout the introduction. However, given that the introduction discusses the unequal power relations that affect graduate students, the intended audience also likely includes graduate professors who are instrumental in determining how academic geographers are made. In a broader sense, the writers may intend the audience to include graduate students and professors of any subject as the writers refer often to "academia," "neo-liberal" university spaces, and "institutional practices."

As we understand it, the question this text seeks to answer is: How does the neoliberal project and the spaces and times it produces within academia play out on our bodies and everyday life experiences as graduate students, specifically academic geography students? This question is first indicated at the end of the first paragraph. The authors believe this is an important question to answer because academia professes an interest in graduate students and faculty having a work/life balance, but it is not set up to produce or support such a balance. Consequently, the only ways to be successful involve adopting ways of doing and being that are white, masculine, and middle-class, which produces productive versus nurturing academic professionals who are required to ignore or subjugate their own well-being to meet the normal standards of academia. The authors do not consider this to be fair, necessary, or the only way things should be.

Headings/Subheadings

I. Introduction

II. Research methods

III. The neoliberalization of academia as an everyday, embodied experience

IV. The logics of neoliberal academic life

    A. The embodiment of neoliberal ideals

    B. Work and life within the neoliberal academy

V. Academic bodies out of place

    A. The "professional" body

    B. The nurturing body

    C. The sick body

VI. Conclusion: Towards some alternatives

The second action we suggested related to noticing macro-level patterns—saving model texts—is just a trick of the trade that can prove very useful for both your immediate and long-term future. Save examples of what you consider to be excellent academic writing, the kind you would like to emulate, in a special place. For example, you might have a folder with a favorite empirical article (e.g., a quantitative, qualitative, or mixed-methods study), a favorite conceptual article (e.g., not an empirical study), a favorite propositional article (e.g., often theory-based), and a favorite response article (e.g., a critical response to previous research). Update this folder with new favorites as your appreciation of "good" academic writing deepens. Also, save examples of writing in which the writer does something well that you know you will also have to do in your own writing. If you know you are planning on doing a study in which you collect interview-based data but you have never written any kind of academic text using that type of data, be on the lookout for a research article or book chapter in which the writer uses interview-based data in ways you find especially effective. Knowing you have models you selected yourself that are readily available can allow you to decide to attempt new forms of writing more comfortably. You will not feel as lost if you have a model or two, and when you get stuck in trying to figure out how to write something up, you can look at your models for guidance and inspiration. See Box 1.2 for our personal stories of how paying attention to different text types as readers helped us as writers.

COMMON MISCONCEPTIONS ABOUT ACADEMIC WRITING

Although the journey to becoming an academic writer is unique and highly individualized, there are some predictable challenges that many new writers

> **BOX 1.2. Preparing for Future Writing through Conscious Reading**
>
> I was once asked to read a published article that was basically an example of conceptual research (i.e., a thorough literature review of what had been done in the field with regard to a specific topic). I found the author's style exceptionally clear and easy to follow. Therefore, I decided to save this particular article as a model for how to write a successful paper that was not empirical but rather just based on a review of the literature. This turned out to be a good idea, as I also found out that in graduate school, often, I was required to write papers that were just reviews of the literature. I returned to this paper time and time again just for inspiration on how to accomplish this task, even though the actual topic of the original paper was nothing like my future papers. Over the years, I have added to my collection of "models" of literature reviews so that now, when I am teaching a student how to do a paper that is only a literature review, I can select from a few I consider appropriate to the current level of academic writing ability the student has.
>
> *—Lauren*
>
> When writing my dissertation, I found the "perfect" journal article amid a gigantic pile of articles I pulled. Instead of feeling like I wanted to skim the article after reading the introduction, this author pulled me into her argument with her passion and urgency about the topic. The article, however, still had the same writing moves I saw in other articles. I saved this article into a file and began keeping an assortment of articles in which I can "hear" the author's voice and feel inspired— because I want my own academic writing to be inspired. Becoming a conscious reader also is embedded in how I take notes. I do not just note the main topics, themes, or take-aways from an article. I also draw a box around phrasing that is creative or especially powerful in delivering a point.
>
> *—Anneliese*

face. One of those challenges is related to previous experience. Many graduate students assume that a past history of succeeding in undergraduate academic writing or workplace writing means they will be automatically or at least easily successful in graduate-level academic writing. This is a myth of epic proportions, and the consequences of believing this myth can be seriously damaging to your self-esteem as both a graduate student and a writer. So two points of awareness we would like for you to embrace are the following:

1. Workplace writing, unless you work as a professor in a university, is not academic writing.
2. The ability to write well in an undergraduate context is not an indicator of the ability to write well in a graduate context.

Why does your writing success in one context not translate to graduate school? Writing is context dependent. What counts as good writing depends on several factors, such as the intended audience/reader, the purpose of the writing, and other things. So, for example, the standards for workplace writing vary from one workplace to another and from one boss to another. In addition, the standards for workplace writing are strongly influenced by the education and capabilities of the people who are intended to read your workplace writing. You could be a great workplace writer in one job and not so great in another simply because your boss or intended readers are different.

The undergraduate experience is similar to the workplace. All teachers have their own expectations about academic writing. Also, undergraduates may write in many different disciplines (e.g., history, psychology, political science, literature) even as they pursue a degree in only one discipline, so they may develop very little understanding of how to write academically within one discipline because they are asked to write in so many different ways.

But does being a "good" writer help at all? Of course, the fact that you have confidence in your capabilities as a writer and probably enjoy it to some extent will definitely help you. It will help you the most if you take the action of accepting from the beginning that graduate academic writing is *not* the same as what you have been doing, and if you become a strategic reader of graduate academic texts in the ways we have already outlined.

Another of the challenges that might pop up for you as you move forward in graduate school is related to unspoken rules. Let's say you are actively and consciously reading. You have picked up several tricks of the trade, and you want to show off your new academic ease in the latest assignment your professor has given you. You put together an academic research essay that sounds just like all of those research articles you have read, right down to the proprietary use of the *we* and *our* pronouns in your introduction and conclusion. You are excited to hear what your professor thinks. You eagerly await the feedback but are floored when your professor critiques the overly confident style of your academic expression and challenges whether you as a student-writer truly have enough knowledge to make such grand and sweeping statements.

"But," you say, "X author did it this way." Yes, X *published* author did, but you are not X, and this work you submitted was not for publication. Welcome to the unspoken rule of academic writing, which states something like the following: *Student academic writers should mimic published academic writers, but they are not allowed to transgress boundaries that more experienced writers may be able to transgress acceptably.* There are some types of academic expression that are too strong or too assertive for student use, and, in fact, many consider them too strong for anyone to use. For example, too much use of *we, our, I,* and *my* is generally frowned upon in academic writing. There are also some permissible assumptions published academic writers can make that student academic writers cannot make. For instance, a published academic writer may be able to use technical terms without definition in his work, whereas a student academic writer would likely need to define those same terms in her own work.

In general, most published academic writers strive to communicate with a rational or neutral tone, which they achieve through the use of both assertive and suggestive language. For example, a phrase such as "The results indicate . . ." is assertive in the sense that it appears that these results are an indisputable fact that the writer is simply reporting. A phrase such as "This finding may be linked to . . . " is suggestive in the sense that the writer is suggesting rather than definitively claiming a link. Student writers are regularly advised to decrease the intensity of their claims by using more suggestive language, such as modals (e.g., *may, might, could*), adverbs (e.g., *perhaps, possibly*), and disclaimers (e.g., *not in all cases, there are exceptions*). See Practice Exercise 1.3 for a practice opportunity related to some of the unspoken rules of writing. You can check your answers in the Appendix.

PRACTICE EXERCISE 1.3. Noticing Some Unspoken Rules of Academic Writing

You have been given two samples of text from the same research article. One sample is from the Introduction, and one is from the Conclusion. Skim both texts and answer the questions that accompany them.

TEXT
(Choi & Miller, 2014, pp. 340, 349–350)

Introduction

Over the past several years, researchers have framed the phenomenon of AAPI's low mental health service utilization in terms of unwillingness to seek counseling. *Willingness to seek counseling* refers to the degree to which individuals are inclined to engage the services of a counselor for academic, vocational, intrapersonal, social, health, or discrimination problems (Gim, Atkinson, & Whiteley, 1990; Kim & Omizo, 2003). Collectively, studies have linked AAPI's willingness to seek counseling to cultural values, stigma, and attitudes toward seeking professional help (Kim, 2007; Ludwikowski, Vogel, &

Armstrong, 2009; Miller, Yange, Hui, Choi, & Lim, 2011; Vogel, Wade, & Haake, 2006; Vogel, Wade, & Hackler, 2007). Therefore, in this study, we tested the ways in which AAPI individuals' adherence to Asian and European American cultural values related to their willingness to seek counseling directly and indirectly through stigma toward counseling and attitudes toward seeking professional help.

Conclusion

Although our findings highlight the ways in which Asian cultural values related to a diminished willingness to seek counseling, it might be more productive to focus on more proximal (and perhaps more malleable) factors such as perceptions of stigma toward counseling rather than attempting to change AAPI individuals' espousal of cultural values (e.g., asking AAPI clients to adhere more strongly to European American values such as independence). In addition, it might be more helpful for clients to explore potential cultural-values-based differences related to seeking counseling. For example, it might be beneficial to help AAPI clients explore how their espousal of Asian and European American cultural values influences their experience of public stigma, stigma by close others, and their own self-stigma toward counseling and how these factors ultimately influence their decision to seek, continue, and/or terminate counseling. Finally, although it is important to acknowledge the impact of cultural values on the counseling process, exaggerated and simplistic distinctions between AAPI and non-AAPI clients could be problematic (Uba, 1994). For example, rather than categorizing AAPI clients as a monolithic racial group and automatically assuming they adhere strongly to Asian cultural values and do not espouse European American cultural values, it would be beneficial to consider the subtle and complex ways in which individuals espouse cultural values and perceive stigma toward counseling.

QUESTIONS

1. Can you find some immediate examples of authors using personal pronouns to establish authorial voice?
2. Can you find some immediate examples of authors using assertive language? When do they use this type of language?
3. Can you find some examples of authors using suggestive language? When do they use this type of language?
4. Now, compare the introduction and the conclusion. Which contains the most assertive language? Which contains the most suggestive language? Why do you think this is?

The reasons that there are unspoken rules of academic writing rest somewhere with the notions of hierarchy and expertise within the academic community. In generations past, most of the people who published academic writing were tenure-track faculty, and, as such, they had earned a certain amount of prestige and writerly discretion in the academic writing culture. Of course, the more published a professor was, the more prestige and discretion he may have been granted within his specific discipline. Thus our best guess (and it is truly a guess) is that, even in today's world, in which graduate students may publish their academic writing, certain manners of expression are allowed or not allowed in direct relation to the writer's need to project a certain amount of prestige in order to be considered worthy of publishing an academic text. However, projecting prestige is not necessary or advisable in graduate-level academic writing. It may have the unintended effect of making the writer seem less rather than more worthy.

How do you obey an unspoken rule—is that not like a dog chasing its tail? Well, it can certainly feel like you are chasing your tail; and it can be quite frustrating because, of course, no one is really going to tell you clearly what to do. We stick by our suggestion that you take action by becoming a strategic reader of academic texts. This will improve your academic writing. The general idea is that the more you read academic writing, the more you absorb how to communicate like an academic writer. The more you absorb, the more you are able to approximate the writing you see in published academic texts. However, as we mentioned earlier, you need to take charge of this absorbing process to ensure that you are moving along the continuum from student-writer to something more than a student-writer. One action we suggest for taking charge of this process is to gently encourage your professors to become more transparent about unspoken rules. You can do this by asking them for what they feel is a "good" model any time they give you a writing assignment. Some professors may offer models when they describe writing assignments, but if professors do not offer a model of a writing assignment, ask them privately or via e-mail if they have a "good" example of the type of writing assignment they wish for students to submit. If they share an example, take time to analyze the sample. You might consider asking yourself questions like the following to increase your understanding of the features that distinguish it:

1. How is this text organized? What are the sections and subsections?
2. What is the purpose of each section and/or subsection?
3. How is the purpose of each section and/or subsection achieved? What content is included? How is the content organized? How is the content expressed from a stylistic perspective?

Each of these questions can help you to understand what counts as good writing to an expert academic writer, namely your professor. If your professor considers this a "good" example, chances are the writing style and skills demonstrated in the assignment are reflective of what matters to that professor and/or in your field.

CHAPTER SUMMARY AND REMINDERS

As we have said in this chapter, we believe there are two fundamental equations that should guide you in developing your academic writing skills: awareness + action = growth and input informs output. We are including a reminder list of awareness and action suggestions from this chapter in Summary Table 1.1 so that you have a handy place to refer to them quickly.

SUMMARY TABLE 1.1. AWARENESS AND ACTION REMINDERS

Be aware . . .	Take action . . .
You will need to take charge of your own journey to becoming an academic writer.	Adopt an attitude of relentless curiosity for figuring out how academic writing is different from other writing.
Academic writing has its own language and style.	Intentionally and consciously expose yourself to as much academic writing language as you can through reading.
You will be asked to read many different types of academic texts. Those texts share some features, but they also each have their own distinctive features.	Actively look for overall macro-level organizational patterns in texts and notice how those patterns compare between texts.
Although you may be or have been a successful writer in many other contexts, you may not experience immediate success as a graduate-level academic writer for various reasons.	Accept that graduate academic writing is a *new* task that will inevitably pose some challenges for you, and strategically use academic reading to inform your knowledge of academic writing.
You are not a published researcher (yet), but your writing needs to move toward approximating the writing of published researchers.	Proactively request models or samples of "good" assignments from your professors so that you can figure out what "good" writing looks like.

CHAPTER 2

Preparing for Writing Success in Your Discipline

As we discussed in Chapter 1, learning how to see texts as an academic writer sees them is a key first step in becoming an academic writer. Incidentally, this is not a one-and-done step, as learning how to see texts through the eyes of an academic writer is a process that may continue for quite some time. However, you do not have to complete this first step before you move on to other steps in the process. Specifically, while you are working on this first step, you can simultaneously begin working on the second step, which is all about learning how to do things the way people in your field do them. We like to think of this step as developing your discipline-specific core. In this step, you work on building the core knowledge base, skills, and strategies for research and writing that are commonly expected of professionals in your field. In other words, you begin learning how to think, act, and communicate like academic professionals in the larger community of practice (CoP) in your field.

Our **awareness focus** for this chapter is on helping you to develop an understanding of how full members of your discipline-specific CoP think, act, and communicate through the written artifacts of your discipline. Our **action focus** includes suggestions and strategies that you can use to actively begin developing the knowledge base, skills, and strategies that will allow you to become more like the full members of the discipline-specific CoP you wish to join.

DISCIPLINE-SPECIFIC COMMUNITIES OF PRACTICE

Unlike most undergraduate programs, graduate programs in social and behavioral sciences, especially doctoral programs, can be seen as loosely based on an apprenticeship model. This means that they are essentially designed to reproduce people who are very much like the professors in the program. Professors are expected to guide graduate students in developing ways of thinking, acting, and communicating that are considered typical in their field. Upon graduation, former students are viewed as reflections of their graduate programs and, more specifically, their advisors. Therefore, professors are like mentors who ensure the growth and longevity of their professional fields by making sure newcomers like you understand and act in accordance with discipline-specific norms.

This mentorship role that professors play can be related to a sociocultural perspective of situated learning known as legitimate peripheral participation (LPP). From this theoretical perspective, the professors in your discipline are part of larger CoP that includes other academic professionals in your discipline (Lave & Wenger, 1991). The people who are long-term members of that discipline-specific CoP, such as your professors, all share some common ways of thinking, acting, and communicating that they learned in the process of *becoming* members of the CoP—that is, they share a discipline-specific core. As the theory explains, they, like you, were once newcomers, and they, like you, had to gradually construct an identity that would allow them to participate as full members in the discipline-specific CoP. They constructed this identity over time, quite probably a long time, through active involvement with the participants, practices, and artifacts of the CoP. Through their active involvement, they learned how participants think and what they think about, what participants do and what they do not do as part of the CoP, and what products the participants produce and what they value in those products.

However, the nature of a true apprenticeship is that one learns primarily by observing and actively participating rather than through direct instruction, which means the apprentice has lots of unobstructed access to the participants, practices, and artifacts of the CoP. This is where graduate school and true apprenticeship may differ, because, unlike true apprentices, graduate students may have limited access to the full members of the CoP (in this case, professors). Graduate students may interact with their professors during class or during office hours, but they may not be observing and working with them 8 hours a day the way apprentices might work with their mentors.

Of course, there are roles for graduate students, such as research or teaching assistantships, that may also provide them with a great deal of fairly unlimited access to full members of the CoP. For example, participating in the practice of collecting data for a professor's study would allow a newcomer to develop a better understanding of how the research process is actualized in their discipline. This type of opportunity may be one that is offered as part of an assistantship, or it may be something that is available if a graduate student proactively seeks it out and volunteers to work with a professor solely for the experience this type of work provides. It is important for graduate students to realize that they can and should seek opportunities that allow them to see firsthand how full members conduct the business of being full members.

In the case of academic discipline-specific CoPs, the primary artifacts are written texts. Graduate students have relatively easy access to the written texts produced by full members of their discipline-specific CoP (however, there are still limitations—e. g., recommendation letters, letters accompanying journal submissions, teaching philosophies). This means that in many ways, for graduate students, written texts are the key to understanding and hopefully joining their discipline-specific CoP. Therefore, as a graduate student, you must use these texts written by full members of the CoP you wish to join as an entry point for developing your discipline-specific academic core. You must use them to figure out how people think, act, and communicate in your field so you can begin becoming more like the full members of your discipline's CoP.

UNDERSTANDING THE THOUGHT AND ACTION NORMS OF YOUR DISCIPLINE

As we have mentioned, the norms of your discipline refer to how people think, act, and communicate in your discipline-specific CoP. Texts written and published by full members of your discipline's CoP are your most accessible key to understanding the norms of your discipline. Written texts can reveal a great deal about how participants in your discipline-specific CoP think and act while simultaneously showing you how they communicate. The natural process for developing your discipline-specific core begins with learning how full members of your discipline's CoP think and what they think about.

Staying "Up" on What's Been Published in Your Field

When you begin a master's program, you may have some knowledge of what topics are valued in your discipline, or you may have none. In fact, many people choose to pursue master's degrees in disciplines that are completely different from the ones they followed for their undergraduate degrees. When you begin a PhD program, you likely have a fairly strong general knowledge base regarding what topics are valued in your discipline, but you may have an incomplete or insufficient understanding of specific issues. Regardless of your degree program, one of the first things you must do to begin developing your discipline-specific core is to figure out what matters in this discipline. To some extent, your coursework will guide you on this path, as professors will naturally select content and materials that are designed to help you understand what matters. They may select broad themes for their classes and have you read discipline-specific artifacts that speak to those themes.

To make the most out of the work your professors have done in selecting materials for you and the work you are doing by reading those materials, you should create a conceptual map for each course you are taking. You can create something fairly simple that has the topic of the course as the center point with broad themes and specific issues radiating outward from it. Ideally, you would create this map in some type of enduring format that would allow you to save and compare the maps from all of your courses. At the end of each semester, you should spend some time reviewing your maps to see how your courses overlap, which themes are repeated, and which issues are addressed under more than one theme. You can use this information to make one integrated conceptual map that illustrates the themes and issues for all of your courses, or you could create some other type of visual organization such as an outline. After each semester, you should update your integrated map so that, by the end of your graduate studies, you have a visual reminder of the entire conceptual framework that was covered by your coursework. See Figures 2.1 and 2.2 for ideas on how to make concept maps. Then follow the instructions in Practice Exercise 2.1 to make your own concept map.

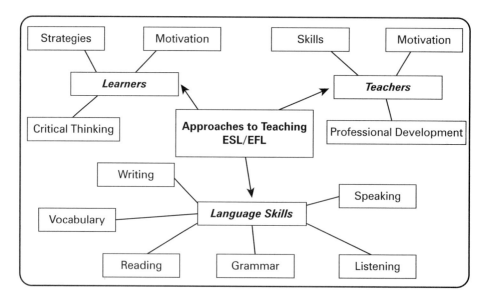

FIGURE 2.1. Abbreviated sample conceptual map for one course.

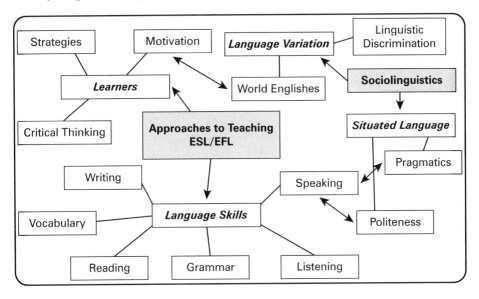

FIGURE 2.2. Abbreviated sample integrated conceptual map linking two courses.

PRACTICE EXERCISE 2.1. Building a Discipline-Specific Conceptual Framework

If you are currently taking a course or have just finished one, find your syllabus and the list of required readings. Try making a conceptual map based on what you see in the topics listed on the syllabus and the topics covered in the readings.

You may find that making the conceptual map forces you to think about the ideas discussed in the course in a new way. You may also find making the map improves your overall understanding of the course.

Try doing it for at least one more course. Then try to see how the topics and ideas of those courses connect.

Now, you may be thinking, "Wow, this is a lot of work—how is any of this going to help my writing?" We agree, it is a lot of work, but the payoff is huge. Research and writing at the graduate level are about connections. New research is based on past research, and a primary purpose of written texts is to interpret the meaning of research findings by explaining how they connect to ideas proposed in previous research. So, in actuality, this conceptual mapping activity has a twofold purpose. On the one hand, you are building a personal mental framework for understanding the relationship between themes and issues on different topics in your discipline, which means that you are developing a knowledge base that will allow you to think more like full members of your discipline-specific CoP. On the other hand, you are developing a practice—the practice of seeing connections between topics and ideas in your discipline—that will not only be conceptually useful to you in your own research but will also bring your way of thinking before you write into closer alignment with what you actually need to do when you begin writing.

Analyzing Research Trends in Your Field

In addition to understanding the topics, themes, and issues that have defined the thinking of your discipline up to now, you also need to develop an understanding of where your discipline is headed. Full members of your discipline-specific CoP are actively engaged in the process of generating new research, and this means that understanding what people in your discipline are thinking about is an ongoing process because the landscape is constantly shifting.

In some of your coursework, you will undoubtedly be exposed to the current research trends and issues in specific areas. However, it is also true that, once established, courses are often taught using the same ideas and many of the same materials for years. Professors may or may not update their courses and the ideas included in them to keep up with changes in the field. Therefore, as a newcomer who wants to become more like a full member, it is up to you to stay up-to-date on what is going on in your field.

The best way to do this is to select two to three of the top journals in your field. Be aware that there are many types of journals from which you can select. There are journals that have an overarching broad focus in an area (e.g., *Psychological Bulletin, Science*), and there are smaller journals that home in on a specific area within your discipline (e.g., *Journal of Specialists in Group Work*). In between these are the journals you should target in your discipline. Anneliese is trained as a counselor and counseling psychologist, so she regularly reads the *Journal of Counseling and Development* and *The Counseling Psychologist,* as they are both geared toward a subdiscipline within the helping professions of counseling and psychology. You will need access to all of the volumes and issues for 3 years prior to the current year. You will also need a blank three-column table with multiple rows (see Table 2.1). We would suggest just setting this up on your computer as an electronic document so that you can cut, paste, reorganize, and modify with ease. Select one of the journals and begin with the volumes/issues from 3 years previous and complete the following steps:

TABLE 2.1. Abbreviated Sample of Analyzing Research Trends		
Categories	**Topics/Themes**	**Articles**
1	Using L2/FL writing as a language learning tool	Ruiz-Funes, M. (2015). Exploring the potential of second/foreign language writing for language learning: The effects of task factors and learner variables. *Journal of Second Language Writing, 28,* 1–19.
2	L2 writers and plagiarism	Davis, M., & Morley, J. (2015). Phrasal intertextuality: The responses of academics from different disciplines to students' re-use of phrases. *Journal of Second Language Writing, 28,* 20–35. Keck, C. (2015). Copying, paraphrasing, and academic writing development: A re-examination of L1 and L2 summarization practices. *Journal of Second Language Writing, 25,* 4–22.
3	ESL writing development and international undergraduates	Knoch, U., Rouhshad, A., Oon, S. P., & Storch, N. (2015). What happens to ESL students' writing after three years of study at an English medium university? *Journal of Second Language Writing, 28,* 39–52.
4	Syntactic complexity in L2 writing	Yang, W., Lu, X., & Weigle, S. C. (2015). Different topics, different discourse: Relationships among writing topic, measures of syntactic complexity, and judgments of writing quality. *Journal of Second Language Writing, 28,* 53–67.
5	L2 writing and feedback	Li, J., Link, S., & Hegelheimer, V. (2015). Rethinking the role of automated writing evaluation (AWE) feedback in ESL writing instruction. *Journal of Second Language Writing, 27,* 1–18. Junqueira, L., & Payant, C. (2015). "I just want to do it right, but it's so hard": A novice teacher's written feedback beliefs and practices. *Journal of Second Language Writing, 27,* 19–36. Willey, I., & Tanimoto, K. (2015). "We're drifting into strange territory here": What think-aloud protocols reveal about convenience editing. *Journal of Second Language Writing, 27,* 63–83.
5a	Editing L2 writing	Willey, I., & Tanimoto, K. (2015). "We're drifting into strange territory here": What think-aloud protocols reveal about convenience editing. *Journal of Second Language Writing, 27,* 63–83.
6	Automatic writing evaluation (AWE) and L2 writing	Li, J., Link, S., & Hegelheimer, V. (2015). Rethinking the role of automated writing evaluation (AWE) feedback in ESL writing instruction. *Journal of Second Language Writing, 27,* 1–18.
7	Teacher beliefs	Junqueira, L., & Payant, C. (2015). "I just want to do it right, but it's so hard": A novice teacher's written feedback beliefs and practices. *Journal of Second Language Writing, 27,* 19–36.
8	Sociocognitive approach to understanding L2 language use	Nishino, T., & Atkinson, D. (2015). Second language writing as sociocognitive alignment. *Journal of Second Language Writing, 27,* 37–54.

(continued)

TABLE 2.1. *(continued)*

Categories	Topics/Themes	Articles
9	Prewriting	Neumann, H., & McDonough, K. (2015). Exploring student interaction during collaborative prewriting discussions and its relationship to L2 writing. *Journal of Second Language Writing, 27,* 84–104.
10	Genre-based approaches to L2 writing	Yasuda, S. (2015). Exploring changes in FL writers' meaning-making choices in summary writing: A systemic functional approach. *Journal of Second Language Writing, 27,* 105–121. De Oliveira, L. C., & Lan, S. W. (2015). Writing science in an upper elementary classroom: A genre-based approach to teaching English language learners. *Journal of Second Language Writing, 25,* 23–39.
10a	Systemic functional linguistics	Yasuda, S. (2015). Exploring changes in FL writers' meaning-making choices in summary writing: A systemic functional approach. *Journal of Second Language Writing, 27,* 105–121. De Oliveira, L. C., & Lan, S. W. (2015). Writing science in an upper elementary classroom: A genre-based approach to teaching English language learners. *Journal of Second Language Writing, 25,* 23–39.
10b	L2 summary writing	Yasuda, S. (2015). Exploring changes in FL writers' meaning-making choices in summary writing: A systemic functional approach. *Journal of Second Language Writing, 27,* 105–121.
10c	L2 thesis writing	Canagarajah, A. S. (2015). "Blessed in my own way": Pedagogical affordances for dialogical voice construction in multilingual student writing. *Journal of Second Language Writing, 27,* 122–139.
11	L2 writing and identity	Canagarajah, A. S. (2015). "Blessed in my own way": Pedagogical affordances for dialogical voice construction in multilingual student writing. *Journal of Second Language Writing, 27,* 122–139. Seloni, L. (2015). "I'm an artist and a scholar who is trying to find a middle point": A textographic analysis of a Colombian art historian's thesis writing. *Journal of Second Language Writing, 25,* 79–99.
11a	L2 writing voice	Canagarajah, A. S. (2015). "Blessed in my own way": Pedagogical affordances for dialogical voice construction in multilingual student writing. *Journal of Second Language Writing, 27,* 122–139.
12	Dialogical pedagogy and L2 writing	Canagarajah, A. S. (2015). "Blessed in my own way": Pedagogical affordances for dialogical voice construction in multilingual student writing. *Journal of Second Language Writing, 27,* 122–139. Fujioka, M. (2015). L2 student–U. S. professor interactions through disciplinary writing assignments: An activity theory perspective. *Journal of Second Language Writing, 25,* 40–58.
13	Intercultural rhetoric	Belcher, D. (2015). What we need and don't need intercultural rhetoric for: A retrospective and prospective look at an evolving research area. *Journal of Second Language Writing, 25,* 59–67.

1. Look through the table of contents to get a sense of what topics and themes are represented in the journal. Notice the types of articles within the journal. Empirical articles are studies of various types, and conceptual articles often describe innovative or emerging ways of thinking within your discipline. There may be other types of articles, such as book reviews, but these are not essential for this activity.

2. Read the abstracts for each article and record the topics and themes you see based on the abstracts in your blank chart, giving each topic or theme its own row. Of course, some articles may appear to touch on more than one topic or theme, and it is fine to include more than one. You may also notice that there are broad, general topics/themes and more specific subtopics/subthemes. Rearrange your table as necessary to record subtopics/subthemes underneath their more general categories. In the end, you will use the numbers column to show the relationship between general topics/themes and subtopics/subthemes (e.g., 1 is a general or unique category, but 1a is a subtopic or subtheme of 1).

3. As you read the abstracts, record some basic bibliographic information about all of the articles that focus on a specific topic or theme (see Table 2.1). Most often, there will be more than one article on each topic or theme in an issue. Again, it is possible that one article may correspond to more than one topic or theme. In those cases, record the article as many times as necessary. (In cases of special issues of a journal, every article may be associated with one topic/theme, but there may also be other subtopics/subthemes addressed within that one topic/theme.)

4. After you finish one issue or volume, repeat the same steps for the next issue or volume, but do not begin a new table. Rather, add to the table that you already have. You may find that you begin to see multiple articles across multiple volumes and issues that are focused on one topic or theme.

5. Continue this process until you have looked at the most recent 3 years of one journal. Then repeat the entire process using a different journal. Again, do not make a new table—just add to the table you have already started. By the time you complete this process using at least 3 years of two different journals, you should have a clear idea of what the current *research trends* in your discipline are.

Table 2.1 reflects only three volumes of one journal. Here are some things we noticed as we prepared this illustration. The first two volumes of the journal we chose produced most of the unique topic/theme and subtopic/subtheme categories. By the time we reached the third volume, most of the articles were fitting in to one of the preestablished topic/theme or subtopic/subtheme categories.

We found that we reorganized the table often as we created it, adding rows below topic/theme categories to create subtopic/subtheme categories.

For this reason, we suggest waiting to add category numbers and letters until the end so you don't have to constantly redo them. We also realized that even more categories could have been created. For example, we did not create categories for the type of research—quantitative or qualitative—or the research approach/technique utilized—longitudinal, case study, think-aloud. Instead, we focused on what the articles were contributing to the knowledge base of the discipline in terms of content. However, we believe adding categories that help you to identify the articles by the type of research they reflect could be very useful for building your understanding of the research practices commonly used in your discipline.

You are probably once again thinking, "This is a lot of extra work!" Yes, we agree that it is, but just as with the conceptual maps you create for your courses, this type of work offers big returns on your investment. By the time you finish this type of analysis, you will know what the current hot topics are in your field. You will have some idea of what the different perspectives on these topics might be. You will also have some idea of the different types of research articles that are published in your field, as well as the different research approaches and techniques that are used in your field. In addition, you may begin to notice who the big names in your field are in relation to specific topics/themes or subtopics/subthemes. In short, you will have gleaned important information from these written artifacts that contributes to developing a strong discipline-specific core. Read Lauren's story of how using this process helped her come up with ideas for her dissertation in Box 2.1, and see what you can learn about topics/themes in your field by completing Practice Exercise 2.2.

PRACTICE EXERCISE 2.2. Understanding the Present and Future of Your Discipline

The most painful part of analyzing research trends using the table we explained is getting started and going through the first few volumes. After the first few volumes, your basic topics/themes and subtopics/subthemes are more or less established. From that point forward, you are generally only reorganizing and occasionally adding new topics/themes and subtopics/subthemes, so let us get you started.

Create a blank table like the one in Table 2.1. Locate the journal you wish to use and commit yourself to following the process of completing the table for at least three volumes or issues of the journal. Once you have gotten that far, we are guessing you will have developed a process for doing it, and you will be inspired to continue by seeing all of the current research that is going on in your discipline.

BOX 2.1. Analyzing Research Trends for Inspiration

There comes a point (or maybe many points) in your graduate studies when you are so inundated with information and ideas that it is very difficult to believe you could ever come up with a new idea that has any value. Yet you know that generating new research is what you are supposed to do if you want to become like your professors. One of the many times I reached this point was when I was trying to come up with ideas for my dissertation. It seemed like every idea I came up with had already been addressed by others. My advisor suggested I look through the previous 5 years of different journals in our field. She did not specify how to do this—she just suggested that doing it might help me to better understand what was currently going on in our field. As I searched, I began creating a table like the one we have asked you to do. At first, I was frustrated by how tedious the task was, but after going through a few issues of the journal, I began to see patterns, and the task became more interesting. Then, after going through several more issues, I began to see all of the different ways research had addressed a particular topic. I could see that sometimes the way one researcher approached a topic was only slightly different from that of another person. I could also see that every topic could be broken down and approached through various subtopics or subthemes. By the time I finished, I could see what had not been addressed for certain topics and where the thinking of my discipline could evolve with respect to specific topics. I felt inspired by all of the possibilities I could see, and I felt more confident about choosing a direction for my own research.

—*Lauren*

Identifying Potential Research Gaps

As we have mentioned, full members of your discipline-specific CoP are involved in actively generating new research, and, ultimately, that is what they would like you to do as well. Coming up with ideas for new research is all about identifying research gaps, and identifying those gaps requires a solid foundation of knowledge about how people in your field think and act.

The identification of a gap is a by-product of your essential disagreement with someone's interpretation of their research findings and/or their research methods. The lack of agreement could be mild—you more or less agree with their ideas, but you think there is more to it, such as additional explanation or evidence that could enhance their interpretation. It could be moderate—you are intrigued by their findings or interpretation, but you are not exactly convinced that their actual findings support their interpretation. Or it could be severe—you see some serious flaws in their research method that you believe invalidate their findings and interpretations. Based on the gap you see, you generate a *new* idea of what issues need to be addressed and/or how to approach those issues.

One important thing to remember about the gap is that it is a perception. In the beginning, it is *your* perception. If *your* perception is not in alignment with how full members of your discipline's CoP think, you will not get very far. In other words, there are unspoken parameters on what is considered a legitimate research gap in every discipline. Fortunately, the artifacts (i.e., research articles) produced by full members generally state the research gap they intend to address, so you have access to an unlimited supply of sample research gaps in your discipline. You can learn the parameters on research gaps in large part by simply analyzing research gaps as they are presented in research articles.

Research gaps are generally presented very near the beginning of a research article, often in the first few paragraphs. The general pattern is that the author begins by introducing a topic and establishing its importance as a research topic by citing several sources that have already established its importance. Then the author points out something that has either *not* been considered about the topic or something that has not been considered *enough* about the topic. This is the research gap. See Practice Exercises 2.3 and 2.4 for practice in identifying research gaps.

PRACTICE EXERCISE 2.3. Identifying and Analyzing Research Gaps

Read each text and answer the questions that accompany it. You can check your answers in the Appendix.

TEXT 1
(Walker-Williams, van Eeden, & van der Merwe, 2012, p. 617)

Women who survive childhood sexual abuse (CSA) often report numerous and varied long-term effects stemming from their experience, which include a range of intra- and interpersonal difficulties (Allen, 2008; Spies, 2006b). Researchers have begun to focus on gaining a better understanding of the risk and protective factors that affect psychological functioning in the face of CSA (Carlson & Dalenberg, 2000). For instance, the trauma of CSA is unique and different to any other childhood trauma. The authors further suggest that CSA victims may develop abuse-related schemas and coping strategies that are adaptive and reflect integration, but which may be "dysfunctional in coping with a world where abuse is not the norm" (Finkelhor & Browne, 1985, p. 533).

Relatively little research has been done on how victims cope with the experience of having been abused sexually as a child and whether or not CSA influences a survivor's coping styles. The identification of coping strategies used by abuse survivors may contribute to a better understanding of factors that protect adaptive functioning and those that put it at risk (Futa, Nash, Hansen & Garbin, 2003).

Questions for Text 1

1. Which sentence(s) refer to the research gap?
2. Why is it considered a research gap according to the authors?

TEXT 2
(Chang, Sharkness, Hurtado, & Newman, 2014, p. 555)

For nearly a decade, governmental agencies (e.g., AAAS, 2001 and National Academy of Sciences, National Academy of Engineering, & Institute of Medicine, 2007) have maintained that the productivity and strength of the U.S. economy will face a serious decline if no significant action is taken to address the racial disparities in the attainment of post-secondary degrees in science, technology, engineering, and mathematics (STEM) fields. The National Science Foundation (NSF, 2009) reported that although African American and Latino undergraduates were just as likely as their White counterparts to enter college with the intention to major in STEM, they were much less likely to earn a degree in those majors. A National Research Council (NRC, 2011) report, Expanding Underrepresented Minority Participation: America's Science and Technology Talent at the Crossroads, stated that most of the growth in the new jobs will require science and technology skills, and that "those groups that are most underrepresented in S&E are also the fastest growing in the general population" (p. 3). Indeed, they write, the proportion of underrepresented minorities in science and engineering would need to triple to match their share in the population. In an effort to achieve long-term parity in the preparation of a diverse workforce, the NAS recommends a near-term goal of doubling the number of underrepresented minorities receiving undergraduate STEM degrees.

As suggested by these reports, the underrepresentation of racial/ethnic minorities is not necessarily attributable to a lack of interest in science fields, but rather to poor degree completion rates. The latter pattern has been well documented. For example, Huang, Taddese, and Walter (2000) found that African American, Latino, and Native American students—or underrepresented racial minorities (URMs)—had lower persistence rates in science and engineering (26%) than their White and Asian American counterparts (46%). A more recent study conducted by the Higher Education Research Institute (2010) found that 33% of White and 42% of Asian American students at a national sample of institutions completed their bachelor's degree in STEM within 5 years of entering college, compared to only 18% of African American and 22% of Latino students. URMs, then, appear to face unique and persistent challenges when moving along the STEM pipeline. However, according to Mutegi (2013), science education research has been unable to explain how science degree achievement is "racially determined." Although students' ability and pre-college preparation are important, steady progress through the STEM pipeline also depends on the types of opportunities, experiences, and support students receive while in college (Chang, Eagan, Lin, & Hurtado, 2011; Espinosa, 2011).

Questions for Text 2

1. Which sentence(s) refer to the research gap?
2. Why is it considered a research gap according to the authors?

TEXT 3
(Bugg, 2013, pp. 1148–1149)

The demise of racially restrictive immigration legislation in the 1970s and a focus on skilled migration has seen Australia undergo profound demographic changes. In the last decade, India has surpassed the UK as the leading birthplace of recent arrivals to Australia, with China close behind [Australian Bureau of Statistics (ABS) 2011]. These demographic changes have resulted in a new Australian religious landscape. Although Christianity has always been predominant in the Australian religious landscape, it has experienced a slow but gradual decline since the time of Australia's federation in 1901. While at the turn of the century 96% of Australians identified themselves as Christians that has decreased steadily and at the last census 61% of respondents identified themselves as Christians (ABS 2011). In contrast, in the last three decades the number of Hindus in Australia has increased sevenfold and the number of Buddhists fivefold (ABS 2011). As these minority religious groups become established, they seek to build permanent places of worship to accommodate their adherents. Australian multicultural policy asserts the right of all citizens to maintain and practice their religion [Department of Immigration and Citizenship (DIAC) 2011]. However, there are frequent conflicts around development applications for minority places of worship and schools (Bugg and Gurran 2011; Dunn 2001). Increasingly, these tensions take place in the rural–urban fringe of Australia's metropolitan areas, a trend that mirrors North America and Europe (for example, Allievi 2010; Echegaray 2010). The study of cities as sites of diasporic religious place making has been extended recently with scholarship on minority religious places of worship in suburban areas (for example, Dwyer, Gilbert and Shah 2012; Marquardt 2006; Waghorne 1999). These claims for space by diasporic religious minorities in exurban areas reflect new patterns of migration, transnational links and social mobility. They also reflect possibilities for the inclusion of minority religious groups in areas that were once socially, culturally and ethnically homogenous.

Questions for Text 3

1. Which sentence(s) refer to the research gap?
2. Why is it considered a research gap according to the authors?

PRACTICE EXERCISE 2.4. Identifying and Analyzing Research Gaps in Your Discipline

- Select one volume or issue of a top journal in your field. Skim through the first few paragraphs of each article until you find the research gap. Ask yourself, "Why is this considered a research gap according to the authors?" Make a note of your answers.
- When you finish one journal, review your answers. What are the most common reasons for identifying something as a gap?
- Make a habit of noticing the research gap and the reason it is considered a gap by the authors in each research article you read. Before long, you will have a very clear understanding of what the parameters are for identifying research gaps in your field.

Getting the Most Out of the Articles You Read

So far, we have focused on ways you can develop your *general* knowledge of how people think and act in your field. By following the suggestions we have outlined up to now in this chapter, you would certainly know what people in your field think about and what they do in terms of research in a general sense. However, obviously, if you truly want to be a full member of your discipline's CoP, you also need to have a more specific, in-depth understanding of *how* they think and *how* they do research. As we explained earlier, you might be able to acquire this understanding by interacting with your professors and actually participating in their research, but as we also explained, you may or may not have those opportunities. That is okay. You will still be able to figure things out. Artifacts in the form of research articles provide great insight into the *hows* of full members' thoughts and research.

Your discipline-specific core is strengthened by repetition, so to get the most out of the research articles you read, you need to develop a systematic approach to reading them, and you need to repeat this approach with each new article you read. This systematic approach includes actually taking some notes—not just highlighting or underlining or cutting and pasting information from a PDF into a document. What we mean by taking notes is actually processing the information you read and communicating it to yourself in a way that reflects your understanding of it.

Although it may be more appealing for reasons of easy record keeping and neatness to take notes using a computer, Mueller and Oppenheimer

(2014) found that taking notes by hand improves note takers' understanding of conceptual information. They hypothesize that the ability offered by computers to transcribe notes in a verbatim fashion may also lead to "shallower processing" of information. When you are reading for academic writing, you are typically reading with the idea in mind that you will be representing and integrating what others have said in your writing. Therefore, you need to engage in deep processing to be absolutely sure that you have an accurate and thorough understanding of their ideas and constructs.

This systematic approach to reading articles also includes reading carefully—not just skimming to find main ideas, results, and interpretations. There is a time and place when skimming is appropriate and helpful, but it is definitely not beneficial when you are trying to develop your discipline-specific core.

So, what is the magic formula for your systematic approach? Unfortunately, this is an unanswerable question. Most graduate students we have talked to (ourselves included) struggle throughout graduate school with what is the *best* way to take notes when reading articles. The *best* way probably depends on what you are trying to accomplish. In this case, we want you to build your in-depth understanding of how people think and act in terms of research in your field. Because of this, we would suggest that your systematic approach should probably include a consideration of the following questions, along with notes on your answers to these questions:

1. What research gap is the article addressing?
2. How does the article intend to address this gap?
3. What are the specific research questions that this article will address?
4. What strands of previous and current research does this article use to create a rationale for its research questions?
5. What kinds of data did the authors collect to answer their research questions and exactly how did they collect them?
6. How did the authors analyze their results?
7. How do the authors interpret their results? According to the authors, what do the results mean with regard to the research question?
8. What do the authors see as limitations in their study?
9. What do the authors see as the implications of this research in terms of either application to real life or directions for future research?
10. What is the authors' overall conclusion?
11. What problems do you see with any aspect of the authors' decision making in this study?

Obviously, the questions we want you to use in your systematic approach are primarily for empirical articles. However, you can just change a few words here and there, and they will likely work for any type of article. After all, the basic premise of research, whether you collect data empirically or not, is to propose a problem and to propose one or more ways of understanding that problem, so all research articles do that in one way or another.

Your next question might be, "How long do I need to follow this systematic approach?" The answer is: As long as it takes for you to develop the discipline-specific core you need to achieve your personal goals. PhD students or master's students who plan to pursue PhDs truly need to develop discipline-specific cores that are like those of full members of the discipline's CoP, so the number of times they need to repeat this approach is greater than it is for those who may be pursuing master's degrees as their terminal degrees.

We can guarantee that following this approach will pay off in the long run. All of the work you do to better understand the artifacts (written texts) of your discipline's CoP will strengthen both your content knowledge and your how-to knowledge. Both of these types of knowledge are crucial precursors to you actually doing research and writing about it.

Reading an Article a Day

In addition to repeating the same systematic approach to the way you read each article, we would also like to suggest that simply reading one new article each day is a straightforward way to build your knowledge base. Of course, you might say, "Do you mean one of the several that I am already assigned to read or something else?" We mean, "Something else!" If you only ever read what you are assigned to read, your knowledge base will grow at a rather slow rate, but imagine if you added just one new article in addition to your assigned ones to each day of the week. Every week, you would read seven new articles in addition to your assigned work. By the end of 1 month, this would be 28–31 articles. Multiply that over the year, and you can easily see how your knowledge base would grow. Reading an extra article each day also increases the speed with which you can read articles, so the more you read, the faster you read. We know students struggle, wondering when they will feel that they have mastered their discipline, but remember that the goal is not to know everything in your field all at once (we do not even know that this is possible!). Your goal is to keep inching ahead in any way you can to consume the literature in your field. Eventually, when you have read deeply enough, you will see that similar concepts are repeated, and you will be able to criticize and synthesize these areas of scholarship. Right now, your goal is to keep reading!

We suggest that you choose these nonassigned articles in one of two ways. Pick a top journal and simply begin reading one article a day from the most recent year of the journal. This will ensure that you are developing an in-depth understanding of your discipline, as well as an in-depth understanding of what that particular journal finds publishable. Or pick a topic that interests you—maybe something you heard about in class or something you discovered when you were analyzing research trends. Find articles related to that topic and read one a day. This will ensure that you are developing an in-depth understanding of your discipline, as well as an in-depth understanding of a topic on which you may wish to conduct research.

We understand that this requires a time commitment that may seem huge, but the rewards will be great and fairly immediate. If you are applying a systematic approach to reading the articles you are assigned for coursework and you are reading an extra article every day to which you also apply a systematic approach, your knowledge base of the whats and hows of your discipline is going to grow exponentially. By the end of just one semester, your discipline-specific core will be significantly stronger than that of a student who is just trying to keep up by understanding the main ideas of readings for class. You will find that you are able to read articles faster, understand them more quickly, use terminology from your field more comfortably, and participate more fully in discussions with your peers and professors. All of this translates into better writing, because all of this prepares you for writing.

UNDERSTANDING THE COMMUNICATION NORMS OF YOUR DISCIPLINE

Up to this point in this chapter, we have focused on how the written texts or artifacts of your discipline's CoP can help you to understand how participants think and act. Of course, the artifacts also represent communication, so they are obviously keys to how full members communicate as well.

As we mentioned in Chapter 1, academic writing is both a culture and a language, but there is a little more to the story than that. In fact, academic writing is simultaneously one culture and many cultures. The many-culture aspect of academic writing is where discipline-specific writing falls. Every discipline, and often even subdisciplines, has its own particular interpretation of exactly how good academic writing is achieved. These interpretations may be codified in language and style guidelines such as APA and MLA, but even if they are, there is still a wide range of variability in what is deemed acceptable and unacceptable.

Some of the reasons for this variability may be attributed to the academic journals that publish research articles. Each journal has author guidelines, and although those guidelines may specify that authors should follow a style such as APA, MLA, or Chicago, the guidelines may also indicate other standards that affect how writing is accomplished. Table 2.2 provides a quick look at excerpts from the websites of three academic journals that represent different disciplines to illustrate how author submission guidelines may influence discipline-specific writing. We talk more about author submission guidelines for peer-reviewed journals in Chapter 9, when we discuss publishing your academic writing.

Notice in Table 2.2 that *TESOL Quarterly* and the *Journal of Counseling Psychology* both specify that authors should follow APA guidelines, but they also both add some other commentary that would necessarily affect how writing is accomplished. For example, *TESOL Quarterly* emphasizes that submissions should be "written in a style that is accessible to a broad readership," which suggests that authors should either avoid technical language or include definitions. It may also suggest that authors should simplify explanations and complex arguments. The *Journal of Counseling Psychology* specifies that submissions should be "concisely written in simple, unambiguous language, using bias-free language," which suggests that authors need to be very attentive to their wording. In this case, the implication may be that the manner in which you express your ideas is just as important as your research or your ideas and could determine whether or not you are published.

TABLE 2.2. Author Submission Guidelines for Peer-Reviewed Journals

TESOL Quarterly

All submissions to *TQ* should conform to the requirements of the *Publication Manual of the American Psychological Association* (6th ed.), which can be obtained from the American Psychological Association. Per APA 6th edition, please note that DOIs are required in references and can be obtained at *www.crossref.org/guestquery*.

TQ prefers that all submissions be written in a style that is accessible to a broad readership, including those individuals who may not be familiar with the subject matter.

Journal of Counseling Psychology

Manuscripts should be concisely written in simple, unambiguous language, using bias-free language. Present material in logical order, starting with a statement of purpose and progressing through an analysis of evidence to conclusions and implications. The conclusions should be clearly related to the evidence presented.

Prepare manuscripts according to the *Publication Manual of the American Psychological Association* (6th edition). Manuscripts may be copyedited for bias-free language (see Chapter 3 of the *Publication Manual*).

American Journal of Education

Manuscripts will be reviewed for the significance of the problem, the originality of the contribution, the cogency of the method and argument, and the crispness and clarity of prose.

List all items alphabetically by author and, within author, by publication year on a separate page titled "References." Do not use APA style.

On the other hand, the *American Journal of Education* specifies that APA should not be used and offers its own detailed guidelines on the website for how to do things such as references. In terms of style, the *American Journal of Education* states that submissions will be evaluated in part based on the "crispness and clarity of prose," which vaguely suggests that authors should be precise and clear in their expression. However, this journal's description is noticeably less detailed than the previous examples, which suggests that this journal may accept a wider variety of writing styles than the other journals.

Given that one of the primary goals of experienced academic writers such as professors is to publish their research in academic journals, it is only natural to assume that their writing styles and beliefs about what is good academic writing in their field are likely shaped by the journals to which they submit their work. In particular, the top journals in a discipline may be the standard bearers for what it means to write well in that discipline. Thus it makes sense to become familiar with the author guidelines for the top journals in your discipline or your subdiscipline.

Familiarizing yourself with author guidelines is fairly easy. We suggest the following five-step process:

1. Ask one of your faculty members, preferably one who works in an area that interests you, what the top journals in the field and, more specifically, her area are. She should be able to give you a list of the ones that she considers most prestigious.

2. Look up each of those journals on the Web. Navigate to the part of the website that includes information for authors.

3. Copy this information into a document and print it out. (Or just print the information if it is already in a PDF.)

4. Once you have the author information for all of the top journals, begin reading through that information carefully. A lot of the information will be the same for all of the journals. This is important, because that information represents the rules of writing that are probably considered normal in your discipline. These are the rules that you also need to learn and follow.

5. If there are guidelines or instructions that you do not understand, these are the writing knowledge gaps that you need to fill. You could attempt to fill these gaps by talking to a trusted faculty member or a fellow student, visiting the campus writing center and consulting with one of their graduate writing advisors, or doing some online research.

If you follow this five-step process, you will definitely have a better idea of what the norms are for your discipline, and you will begin the process of developing discipline-specific core writing skills. You will be learning how to write like the experts by developing an understanding of the processes they go through to publish an article. As a bonus, you may be able to understand your professors' commentary on writing better because you may recognize that their commentary is related to author submission guidelines. For example, if your professor comments that your language is not "crisp" enough, you will at least understand why he is making this comment and why the concept of "crispness" matters.

Another factor that affects discipline-specific writing is the type of research discussed. For example, whether you are writing up a quantitative or a qualitative study may affect the writing norms of your discipline. Writing up quantitative research tends to result in more formulaic writing in which specific types of sentences and phrasing are common. On the other hand, qualitative write-ups have more variability and may even become almost story-like in their delivery.

Texts written and published within your discipline's CoP provide an endless supply of information on how to communicate like a full member because they provide an endless supply of examples of how communication is accomplished. For example, a novice writer might use the personal pronoun "I" and conclude that this is acceptable. It may be acceptable within your discipline and/or area of study; however, we would caution that novice writers should check with professors before assuming that student authors are allowed to use personal pronouns in this manner. Ultimately, becoming a conscious reader and building a personal library of model research articles, as we discussed in Chapter 1, can help you pick up the style of expression preferred in your discipline naturally and easily. Whenever you feel yourself struggling with how to express an idea, find an article in your field and look for model sentences and phrasing that can help you articulate your ideas within the norms of your discipline.

PREPARING YOURSELF FOR THE JOURNEY OF "BECOMING"

Although we have mainly focused on the external nature of your journey to becoming a member of your discipline's CoP—that is, learning how full members think, act, and communicate—there is also an internal component to building a discipline-specific core. The internal component is all about getting very clear and honest with yourself about any gaps in your own preparation to begin the journey and doing something about those gaps. Some of the most common gaps are: not being familiar with the general style guidelines used in your discipline (e.g., APA, MLA, *Chicago*), not having strong library research skills, not having strong general writing skills, and not having a strong understanding of the research writing process. All of these gaps can create obstacles for you in the journey of becoming like your professors. To address these gaps, we suggest the following:

• Find out what academic style system is preferred in your discipline (e.g., APA, MLA, *Chicago*), buy the manual, and read it. Some of them, such as APA, actually offer ancillary workbooks in which you can practice the concepts discussed in the manual. Buy the workbook and work through it. The process is potentially boring and tedious, but ultimately you will have acquired a basic stylistic knowledge of the writing conventions of your field that will set you apart from other graduate students who do not take this step. Do this in the beginning, such as in the first semester of your graduate studies. Professors expect you to know these things, but they are not necessarily going to teach you these things.

• Use campus resources to strategically improve your writing. If, for example, you do not know how to use the university library but you need to do library research, find out what workshops are offered by the library so you can obtain the skills you need. If you are concerned that you may not be integrating sources into your writing appropriately or if you are unsure about plagiarism, go to the university's writing center and set up an appointment with a tutor. You could even set up an appointment to work with a tutor every week on the same assignment throughout the semester until it is finished. Libraries may also provide access to citation software such as Zotero, Endnote, or Mendeley. Whether or not the library provides access to the software, it is likely that the search tools hosted by the library have compatibility with one or more types of citation software. Investing time early in your graduate studies to learn how to use citation software will be a great time saver as you progress in your studies. Check with your campus library to find out what software they offer and/or support. Also, check to see whether they provide any type of online or in-person tutorials for learning how to use citation software. If they don't offer tutorials, look online, as there are plenty of free resources that explain how to use citation software.

• Understand your unique challenges as an academic writer. Perhaps punctuation has just never been your strong suit. Okay, that is fine, but hire an editor to look at your academic writing assignments before you submit them. This will mean that you need to get things finished earlier than normal and spend extra money, but it will also ensure that you are submitting academic writing that will be carefully considered for the overall quality of its ideas rather than discounted for its sloppy mechanics. However, before you hire an editor, please verify that using an editor is permitted in your department. Some graduate programs may consider writing without outside assistance part of your professional training.

• Improve your time-management skills for completing assignments that must be done over long periods of time. Last-minute writing really, really does not work in graduate school. Yes, it often does work in undergraduate classes, but no, your professors will not let you get by with it in graduate school. Graduate classes typically require lots of reading, lots more than any undergraduate class you took. These classes also require lots of writing, and the expectations for the quality of that writing are much higher than they were for undergraduate classes. Remember, as a graduate student, professors are looking at you as a future potential colleague in their field. When you submit writing that is at best undergraduate in quality, their protective instincts for their field go up. They most assuredly do not want to let someone become a colleague who is not able to communicate in writing the way one should in their field. You need to carefully plan your time and consider how long each step of your writing assignment will take. As a graduate student, you are expected to have professional time-management skills. You are expected to get things done on time. You are also expected to know if you are not going to get things done on time well before they are due, and you are expected to communicate that clearly and directly with your professors well before the due date. It is likely that they will work with you even if they do express disappointment. Importantly, please factor in a longer amount of time than you think you will need for the revision process—your own revision process as you write and the one that your readers might request after they read your writing. Revisions in graduate writing can be quite extensive and time-consuming. Your readers and/or your own inner writing critic may ask you to completely rewrite things that your writer-self considered complete. For example, Grant and Pollock (2011) found that winners of the *American Management Journal* Best Article Award rewrote their introductions 10 times. Clearly, if published professionals are rewriting their own introductions 10 times, the number of times less experienced writers may need to rewrite their own work is at least as much but probably much higher.

• Strategize assignments with your professors. They have office hours, they have e-mail, and they probably will even talk with you after class. If you are working on the plan for your writing assignment, send them a written version of your plan and ask for feedback. They may be able to see a logic error or two in just a basic plan that will save you hours. They may also be able to recommend sources or simply provide you with encouragement.

CHAPTER SUMMARY AND REMINDERS

Throughout this chapter, we have emphasized the idea that you as a graduate student are engaged in a process of becoming a member of your discipline's CoP and that part of that process is developing your discipline-specific core. Learning the whats and hows of full members' thoughts and practices in your CoP are a necessary part of your development as a writer in your discipline, because we believe a majority of writing is actually not writing—it is all the things you do before you write. Summary Table 2.1 lists the awareness and action suggestions we have made throughout this chapter.

SUMMARY TABLE 2.1. AWARENESS AND ACTION REMINDERS	
Be aware . . .	Take action . . .
Joining the CoP of any discipline requires you to understand how full members think, act, and communicate.	Develop the ability to see connections between ideas in your field, because this will allow you to build a conceptual framework similar to that of a full member of your discipline's CoP.
Understanding the past, present, and future of a discipline's ways of thinking is fundamental to becoming a member of that discipline.	Stay up-to-date on where your discipline is headed by familiarizing yourself with the current research trends in your field's top journals.
Learning the parameters of what qualifies something as a viable research gap is essential for understanding how members of your discipline think.	Notice research gaps in every study that you read and develop your ability to identify research gaps in current research trends.
Becoming like a full member requires you to know not only what members do but how they do it.	Discover the hows of your discipline by committing to careful and regular reading of full members' written texts.
Full members of a discipline-specific CoP follow very similar strategies for communicating their ideas in writing.	Notice and mimic the style of communication that you see in full members' written texts.
The norms of discipline-specific writing may be standardized to some extent, but they may also vary according to the stylistic preferences of different academic journals.	Familiarize yourself with the stylistic preferences of the top journals in your field and seek assistance with any elements of writing style that are unfamiliar to you.

CHAPTER 3

Developing Your Own Writing Identity

Finding your own academic writing voice is somewhat like finding your place in your discipline-specific CoP. It is an ongoing process that may continue well beyond the end of your graduate studies as you continue to integrate the thought, action, and communication norms and possibilities of your discipline. The process may end once you discover a particular research niche and begin to regularly produce written texts for your discipline's CoP that are accepted for publication. However, for many researchers, the process of finding their own voices continues throughout their careers as they integrate new ideas and changes in their field to their own established ways of thinking, acting, and communicating.

Our **awareness focus** for this chapter is to help you to develop an understanding of what academic writing voice is and why it matters. Our **action focus** includes suggestions and strategies you can use to engage in the process of finding your own academic voice.

ACADEMIC WRITING VOICE: WHAT IS IT, AND WHY DOES IT MATTER?

Up to now, we have focused on how you need to learn to be more like other people—academic writers in general (Chapter 1) and full members of the CoP in your discipline more specifically (Chapter 2). You may be somewhat disheartened by the prospect of graduate students like you being forced to replicate their mentors and their discipline-specific CoPs. If that were all there was to it, we agree it would be disappointing and demotivating. However, as Lave and Wenger (1991) explain, CoPs need new members who can both reproduce the norms of the CoP and challenge them. They need the fresh and unique perspectives of newcomers to avoid stagnation and ultimately the dissolution of the CoP. So, yes, as a graduate student, you are expected to *conform* to the norms of your field, but you are also expected to *propose* new, unique interpretations of those norms. To fulfill these somewhat contradictory expectations, you will need to find your own academic writing voice.

At first glance, the term *academic writing voice* seems to imply something about a writer's communication style. However, style is only one part of academic writing voice; there's much more to it. Academic writing voice is in its broadest sense the unique pattern of choices a research writer makes regarding content, approach, and expression. This pattern of choices functions as the researcher's writing identity. That is, this pattern becomes the face or voice of the researcher within her discipline-specific CoP. Others in the CoP come to know the researcher not as a person but as a voice. Like a person, a voice has unique qualities, and in fact, in the academic world, it is highly important that a researcher strive through her choices to create a distinctive voice.

As you may recall from Chapter 2, newcomers to a discipline-specific CoP are learning how to become like full members by learning how they think, act, and communicate. In essence, newcomers are learning the collective voice of their discipline's CoP. We referred to this as learning the norms. However, these norms should not be interpreted as fixed boundaries. Rather, they should be thought of as preferences that point to possibilities.

For example, a norm—such as which term, *subject* or *participant,* should be used to represent the people who take part in a research study— may at a given point in the history of the discipline have what appears to be a decisive answer (e.g., use the term *subject*), and this answer may even be codified in the style guidelines of the discipline. Nonetheless, over time there may be a growing number of newcomers and full members who are exposed to new perspectives on the use of the term *subject.* These new and continuing research writers may choose to use the term *participants* instead of *subjects,* thereby treating the norm not as a fixed boundary but as a preference that points to the possibility of change. In effect, these writers are making a choice about their own writing voices that is also an attempt to change the collective voice of their discipline.

In the beginning, their use of the term *participant* might result in requests for modification from professors and editors to replace the term *participants* with *subjects.* However, these requests may also result in information exchanges whereby those requesting the change become more informed about the reasons the writers wish to use the term *participants.* Some of those professors and editors who requested changes may become convinced by writers' explanations that the use of the term *participants* is preferable, and they may begin to allow it. Over time, the number of professors and editors who accept the use of the term *participants* may grow to such a majority that the norm itself changes and is codified in the style guidelines of the discipline, thereby changing the collective voice of the discipline. Thus discipline-specific norms can be used as points of departure for making choices outside of the norm.

A researcher's writing voice reflects the collection of choices he has made at these points of departure, and each researcher strives to make a unique collection of choices so that he is both part of the collective voice and distinctive within the collective voice. The choices that become a research writer's voice include the following general and specific points of departure, among others: content, as reflected through topic; approach, as reflected through perspective, research methods, and research techniques; and expression, as reflected through syntax, word choice, grammar choices, and even punctuation. The research writer may choose to remain within the norm on some of these points, to slide slightly outside the norm on others, and to slide more significantly outside the norm on others. The goal of every research writer is to find a particular configuration of settings on these points of departure that establishes the individuality of his voice within the CoP.

As we discussed in Chapter 2, all research begins with a research gap, and choosing that gap is part of finding an academic writing voice. Choosing a gap is related to both choosing content or topic and choosing an approach. Newcomers must learn what general topics are considered worthy of research in their disciplines, and they must look for specific topics within those general ones that will offer them the opportunity to make unique contributions. It is a bit like looking for tiny crevices in a sidewalk— newcomers are looking for openings in the CoP that they can fill with their research and new ideas.

To illustrate, in the field of counseling, a newcomer would notice that such topics as the counselor–client relationship, clients' presenting issues, and theories of counseling are general topics that are deemed worthy of study in the discipline-specific CoP. A newcomer who wants to distinguish her voice through her choice of research topic might choose to work in the area of power differentials in the counselor–client relationship, because this is a crevice in the general topic of the counselor–client relationship that currently needs to be filled. It is an emerging topic that a newcomer could choose that would distinguish her writing voice through choice of content.

Choices related to approach are also related to finding a writing voice and a research gap. Three points of departure—perspective, research methods, and research techniques—contribute to choosing an approach. All behavioral and social science disciplines include a variety of perspectives or points of view regarding research in general and specific topics. Newcomers may choose to use an established perspective to research a new topic in order to distinguish their writing voices from those of others, or they may choose to use a new perspective to research an existing topic.

For example, general research perspectives are one point of departure that may help newcomers find a unique writing voice. General research

perspectives include positivist, postpositivist, and poststructuralist perspectives. One of the ways in which these perspectives are distinguished
is in the way each perspective views the idea of truth or fact. A positivist
perspective holds that there is one truth that can be discovered through
the application of specific research procedures. A postpositivist perspective
maintains that there are multiple truths that are all equally valid (i.e., there
are simultaneous truths). A poststructuralist perspective views truth as
something that is interpreted through the lens of privilege and oppression.
In other words, forces that have shaped the interpreter's view of the world
influence truth. A newcomer to a discipline or topic that favors a positivist
approach could choose to focus on a topic that is relatively common in the
discipline but from a postpositivist perspective, thereby creating a writing voice that simultaneously upholds the collective voice and distinguishes
itself from that voice.

Just as the choice of research perspective is a point of departure that
contributes to establishing a newcomer's approach, so too is the choice of
research methods and research techniques. In fact, an academic writer's
voice is heavily influenced by the research methods and techniques he
chooses. For instance, a newcomer who chooses qualitative research as his
method in a field that is predominately quantitative will most certainly
not only stand out as unique but will likely also face significant challenges
from those who evaluate his writing due to the ideological differences this
choice represents. If this same newcomer decides to push the boundaries
of his mostly quantitative discipline even further by selecting ethnography,
and more specifically autoethnography, as his technique, his voice will be
significantly different from the voices of those in the field. In a case such as
this one, in which the newcomer has chosen to diverge from the collective
voice in so many ways, the newcomer's voice may actually struggle to find
an audience in his discipline because the voice he has created is so different
from that of the discipline.

As we alluded to earlier, academic writing voice is related to a writer's
style of expression. Aspects of style include syntax, or how sentences are
structured; word choice; grammar choices; and even punctuation. Although
communicating ideas in acceptable ways within a discipline is paramount
to becoming a full member, it is also important for writers to find their
own style. A writer's style is usually what makes you like or not like reading
his research. You might think of style like personality. The choices writers make, from how long their sentences are to the transition words they
choose to use to their use of punctuation marks such as semicolons and en
dashes, are like personality traits. We are drawn to some writers' styles just
as we are drawn to some people's personalities. When we like a writer's
style, we also generally find his arguments easier to understand and more
persuasive. Try your hand at comparing authors' styles in Practice Exercise
3.1 by looking at excerpts from Kim (2014) and from Hawkins, Manzi,
and Ojeda (2014). You can compare your answers to ours in the Appendix.

PRACTICE EXERCISE 3.1. Noticing and Comparing Writers' Styles

Read through the excerpts in the following illustration. As you read, think about which text you prefer and consider the reasons for your preference. Try to answer the following questions after you read.

1. Is your preference related to content, approach, or expression?
2. Is one of the texts easier for you to understand and follow? If yes, what makes that text easier? Notice the words and phrases highlighted in each text.
3. Each text contains at least two patterns in the writers' stylistic choices. What are the patterns?

TEXT 1

[1]Little research exists, however, to document the realities of the transition to college for Chinese and Korean immigrant students. [2]The educational success of Asian American students, considered as a homogenous group, often conceals the diverse experiences and complex challenges arising between and among Asian immigrant student ethnic groups, resulting in a lack of specific research and immigrant-targeted best practices. [3]Therefore, in this study, I sought to fill that gap by examining how Chinese and Korean immigrant students negotiate their parents' expectations, thus illuminating in greater detail the role that parents play in the college-going processes of their children. [4]More specifically, I examined how the educational experiences of 1.5 generation Chinese and Korean immigrant college-age students differed by socioeconomic background and ethnicity. [5]The term "1.5" specifies students who immigrated as children or youth, in contrast to adult immigrants (first-generation) or youth who were born

TEXT 2

[1]Below, we briefly outline our research methods and then highlight some of the literature that has inspired us to pursue this research. [2]Subsequently we examine some of the themes emerging from this project including the way in which the pressures of the neoliberal academy are normalized in the lives of the graduate students that participated in this research project, the experiences of these students working within a meritocracy, and the blurring of work and life under a competitive, neoliberal model. [3]Our work draws from critical analyses of neoliberalism's capacity to produce particular subjects (e.g., Dean, 1995; Rose, 1993). [4]It seeks to contribute to the question of how the neoliberal project, its practices and discourses, translates into particular geographies (see Peck and Theodore, 2012 and Castree et al., 2006), focusing particularly on the intimate, bodily scale. [5]Taking this into account, we then illustrate the ways in which the neoliberal university interacts with particular bodies that are deemed *out of place*. [6]Here we

in the United States with immigrant parents (second-generation). [6]I was particularly interested in 1.5 generation immigrants because these students often face the challenges of reconciling cultural differences and adjusting to the educational system of their host country, demonstrating different adaptation experiences compared to either their first- or second-generation counterparts (Hurh, 1990; Lee & Cynn, 1991; Lee, 2001; Rumbaut & Ima, 1988).

follow Tim Cresswell's (1996) and Linda McDowell's (1999) argument on how gendered relations play an important role in the ways in which particular bodies are assigned to particular spaces, deeming certain bodies—e.g., sexualized bodies, sick bodies, pregnant bodies, non-heterosexual bodies, etc.—as bodies "out of place." [7]This mutual coding of bodies and neoliberal spaces is of particular importance to us as we seek to better understand the material and symbolic places we are assigned within the political landscapes of academia. [8]In particular, we address the pressures students feel to embody white, masculine and middle-class subject positions. [9]We discuss the production of productive bodies as opposed to nurturing ones, and the perceived impacts that working in the neoliberal university has over health and general wellbeing. [10]We conclude with some thoughts on negotiating and generating alternatives to these processes through our ongoing 'Lives in the making' project.

Finding an academic writing voice is a necessary rite of passage for all newcomers. All newcomers must develop a writing identity or voice, which they do through the choices they make regarding content, approach, and expression. Importantly, newcomers must strive both to conform to the collective voice of their disciplines and to distinguish their own voices. Voices that conform too much or differ too greatly may go unheard (i.e., unpublished). Therefore, it is imperative that as a newcomer, you understand the choices available to you and the potential consequences of those choices.

FINDING YOUR OWN ACADEMIC WRITING VOICE

Finding your own academic writing voice is a process that begins early on in your graduate training. You are trained and encouraged to adopt a critical perspective on all that you hear and read. Your professors want you to critique and synthesize the research you read. They want to know that you are able to discern the strengths and the weaknesses of research in your discipline. They want to know that you can imagine and propose ways of improving upon perceived weaknesses. They want to know that you have opinions that are based on an in-depth understanding of your field and the particular research study in question.

In the beginning, this kind of critique may be hard for you, as your limited knowledge base may prevent you from the kind of in-depth understanding that is required. However, assuming that you actively attempt to build your knowledge base of the thought and practice norms of your discipline, you will begin to notice what types of thoughts, practices, and communication styles appeal to you most and least. You will begin to notice that some research seems more credible to you than other research, and you will begin to develop the ability to pinpoint reasons for this. You will notice that not all research in your field is the same, and you will begin to see that within your field, perspectives on the same issue may be widely divergent or even completely contradictory. You will notice that you may feel more aligned with some perspectives than others for a variety of reasons, including personal reasons. You will notice that the quality of research writing in your field may also vary. Some texts may be clearly and engagingly explained, whereas others are more esoteric and less interesting to you. All of this is part of the process of discovering which types of academic writing voices you prefer.

Of course, finding your own academic writing voice is easier the more familiar you are with the scholarship in your discipline. This can make the task of finding your own voice seem overwhelming, because there is so much to know. You may feel that you are supposed to "know it all" when it comes to your discipline. We think about this a little differently. We agree that it is important to be on the path where you are learning more and more about your discipline. We also strongly believe it is important for you to critically consume the literature of your discipline. However, many students focus so much on knowledge acquisition that they forget to have opinions on what they are reading and consuming in their discipline. This is a tricky situation, as the whole point of seeking an advanced degree is not only to expose yourself to new ideas and new ways of thinking about your discipline but also to be an active contributor to those very same new ideas and new ways of thinking in your field. As we mentioned earlier, you have to both fit in and stand out.

Our ideas about fitting in have already been discussed in Chapters 1 and 2, so let us talk about how to stand out or, more specifically, how to find your own academic writing voice. Don't think about the last article you read or the last research lecture you attended. Instead, think back to the last debate you got into—and make sure it was a lively debate (not an argument) in which strong and passionate perspectives were shared. Maybe this debate was with a colleague, partner, family member, or friend. Think back to this debate, and in particular, think about the choices you made. What points did you choose to focus on in the debate? What evidence did you choose to use in support of your points? How did you choose to express your ideas to make them as convincing as possible? In other words, how did you try to make your argument stand out?

Debating involves strategic decision making, and so does academic writing. In both debating and academic writing, the general goal is to persuade the audience to consider your argument as a valid and worthy point of view; it is understood that you may not be able to persuade the audience to agree with you, so that is generally not your goal. Your choices affect your audience's willingness to consider your point of view by either opening or closing the door on that willingness. This is obvious in face-to-face debates. We know, for example, that a condescending or angry tone of voice will most likely close the door. The same is true of writing. The voice you choose to use will either draw your readers in or send them packing. Therefore, you want your academic writing voice to reflect your enthusiasm, passion, understanding, and engagement. Look over the following examples and notice how each makes you feel as a reader:

SEND-'EM-PACKING EXAMPLE

There has been little research on the experience of youth in the language and literacy field.

DRAW-'EM-IN EXAMPLE

We argue that in the context of literacy teaching and learning in contemporary United States, the weak and underrepresented includes generations of youth who have been underserved or completely marginalized by and through language and literacy in the classroom. (Jones & Rainville, 2014, pp. 183–184)

The send-'em-packing example is not a bad sentence. It is concise and gets to the point, which are certainly skills we need to have in our academic writing toolbox. But, let's be honest, it is a boring sentence that could have been written by anyone—it does not have a personality. You know the general topic that this author intends to address, but you do not really have any idea of the author's voice from this sentence.

However, the draw-'em-in example provides much more insight as to the authors' voices. It provides more specific information on the topic and points of view that will be discussed. It also reflects the authors' enthusiasm, passion, understanding, and engagement in the topic. These authors have points of view that they are passionate about, so passionate in fact that they are willing to "argue" for these points of view. For example, they believe that U.S. youth should be counted as part of society's "weak and underrepresented," and they believe that youth have been "underserved or completely marginalized" by language and literacy practices. Readers are likely to be provoked to read their text by the energy in these authors' voices. These authors are not inviting readers into a ho-hum text; they are inviting them into a debate.

Finding your own enthusiastic, passionate, understanding, and engaged voice takes time, but all of that reading we asked you to do in Chapter 2 can help you. As you do all of that reading, think about what types of academic writing *inspire* you. How will you know if you are inspired?

- You will enjoy reading the text.
- You will feel excited by the ideas in the text.
- You will have questions about the ideas in the text not because something wasn't explained but because you feel genuine curiosity.
- You will spontaneously begin thinking about how the ideas in the text connect to your own ideas or ideas from other texts.
- You will find the text easy to read and feel like the author is "speaking your language."
- You will find yourself saying, "Yes, yes, yes," as you read the text because you can clearly see how everything in the text fits together and makes "perfect sense."

We think of these inspiring voices we find through reading as virtual mentors. We usually do not know the people behind these voices, but the identities they communicate through their writing in some way guide us. Look for one of your virtual mentors in Practice Exercise 3.2.

PRACTICE EXERCISE 3.2. Finding Inspiration in the Voices of Other Writers

Select an article in your discipline or an area you know something about that meets the criteria for *inspiring* you. Answer the following:

- What inspires you about this article? Is it the topic, the approach, the research method, the research techniques, the writing style, or some combination of these factors?
- In what ways is the author of this article following the norms of her field? In what ways is she sliding outside those norms?
- How did the author of this article draw you in? How did the author keep you interested and engaged?
- What aspects of this author's voice would you like to emulate? Why?

Although looking for inspiration in others' texts is useful and may be the safest route to finding a voice—safe because you are patterning yourself after someone who has a voice that is already accepted in your discipline—we think you can also look internally for your inspiration. It is easy in graduate school to become so focused on learning how others think, act, and communicate that we forget ourselves. We forget we have personal preferences, motivations, and interests that drive us. Finding your own writing voice is sometimes a matter of allowing the personal to influence our writing choices. Communicating with passion, enthusiasm, understanding, and engagement is much easier when we are actually personally invested in our communication. Therefore, connecting aspects of our personal beliefs and interests to the choices we make for writing can result in a marked change in the quality of our writing voice and our own appreciation for that voice.

For example, a major challenge of academic writing is figuring out what you want to say about a particular topic. For newcomers and members alike, this can be simultaneously the most exciting and frustrating aspect of academic writing. In terms of excitement, maybe this is a topic near and dear to your heart, or maybe the topic is something you have been passionately building toward for a long time. However, you may feel frustrated because you are not quite sure how to go about pursuing your passionate personal interest in a way that connects with what has been written about or studied in the field before. Or you may feel like everything on your topic has already been studied. When this happens, you need to create your own "aha!" moment.

To provide an idea of what this looks like in real life, Anneliese studies the resilience of transgender people. She did not enter graduate school knowing she wanted to study this topic. She did enter graduate school with a passionate personal interest in social justice and community service. These interests were related to her upbringing and the faith in which she was raised, Sikhism. She also entered graduate school with some life experiences that made her especially interested in helping the world to be a kinder place for people who were typically marginalized. She had personally experienced a lot of bullying growing up as a person of color in the South with a turban-wearing Indian dad and white mom. She spent her formative teenage years hanging out in the gay bars of New Orleans, where she learned about loving and accepting herself from the many LGBTQ friends she found there.

Once Anneliese began to explore the topics of her field, she realized that two topics—resilience and transgender people—particularly interested her. Both of these topics connected with profoundly important experiences in her life, so she had a great deal of passion for these topics. She had been exploring transgender identity development in her coursework and realized there was a good deal of work that spoke to the discrimination transgender people experienced in society. However, she felt frustrated as she explored the idea of transgender resilience because she would see the word *resilience* quite a bit in literature that was *not* about transgender people. There was a bunch of literature, for instance, on the resilience of children from historically marginalized communities. She was personally moved by the concept of resilience but could not find the connections she wanted to see with transgender people. How could she bridge the gap between these two literature bases of transgender identity development and resilience in children? How could she integrate her personal interests with the existing research in the field? She held these questions for quite a while (and felt frustrated for quite a while). Then, one day she had her "aha!" moment. The "bridge" was that she was not so much interested in the individual resilience of transgender people but was very much interested in, passionate about, and excited to write about their resilience to actual societal oppression, which connected to her personal interest in social justice. This mixture of excitement and frustration has now led her to spending over 15 years studying transgender resilience.

So, if we do a little bit of analyzing of what exactly set her up for this "aha!" moment, you can see how the tension between the personal and the professional led her to frustration and how frustration led her to thinking about, exploring, and dissecting how ideas that were personally meaningful to her fit into the larger literature. The key to exploring this tension and ending up with an "aha!" moment is leaning into our curiosity. Curiosity is that key because it taps into our intrinsic motivation. It is an emotion that motivates us to persevere in overcoming obstacles because we see the ultimate goal as personally valuable. Therefore, finding your personally motivating curiosity can be very helpful for finding your own writing voice.

The good news is that curiosity is a natural part of being human! In academic writing, we want to support you in reconnecting with that curiosity. To encourage you in this reconnection, here is this pretty famous quote by Rainer Maria Rilke from *Letters to a Young Poet* (1934):

> Try to love the questions themselves as if they were locked rooms or books written in a very foreign language. Do not search for the answers, which could not be given to you now, because you would not be able to live them. And the point is to live everything. Live the questions now. Perhaps then, someday far in the future, you will gradually, without even noticing it, live your way into the answer. (Letter 4)

So, hold on to your curiosity. Do you remember the reason you decided to pursue higher education? Rilke would want you to hold on to that feeling. Remember the last time you Googled something, and you just kept reading deeper and deeper into the topic of your search? We would say that was your curiosity at work. Remember the time you learned the rules of a new game, felt confused, and were still excited to start the game? This is your curiosity at play. You might even say that curiosity is the hallmark emotion of all academia and other formal and informal levels of study. Curiosity is one of your BFFs in academic writing, so connect with your curiosity and use it to find your voice. Use Practice Exercise 3.3 to get you started.

PRACTICE EXERCISE 3.3. Intentionally Setting Yourself Up for an "Aha!" Moment

Answer the following questions:

- What are a few themes, topics, or subtopics in your field that you find personally interesting?
- How is your interest in these themes/topics/subtopics related to your personal experiences?
- What do you know about these themes/topics/subtopics based on personal, lived experience?
- What would you guess the literature in your field might say about these themes/topics/subtopics?
- How might you be able to bridge your personal interest in these themes/topics/subtopics with the existing research on them? What might you be able to find out that would be personally meaningful to you through this research?

In addition to looking for virtual voice mentors through your reading and looking inside your own personal experiences for voice guidance, you can also use writing as a way to work on finding your voice. Now, we realize that using writing to find your writing voice seems like a contradiction in terms, but you can actually discover your writing voice through writing. The exact term for this type of writing is *writing to learn*. Fulwiler and Young (2000) describe how writing can allow writers to learn from themselves in the following manner:

> We write to ourselves as well as talk with others to objectify our perceptions of reality; the primary function of this "expressive" language is not to communicate; but to order and represent experience to our own understanding. In this sense language provides us with a unique way of knowing and becomes a tool for discovering, for shaping meaning, and for reaching understanding. For many writers this kind of speculative writing takes place in notebooks and journals; often it is first-draft writing, necessary before more formal, finished writing can be done. Finally, writing is a value-forming activity, a means of finding our voice as well as making our voice heard. The act of writing allows authors to distance themselves from experience and helps them to interpret,

clarify, and place value on that experience; thus, writers can become specta-tors using language to further define themselves and their beliefs. (p. x)

Writing to learn includes free-form writing, lists, notes, memos, and other forms of writing that reveal ideas you never even knew you had. We think writing-to-learn strategies like the following can help you find your voice.

Writing Prompts

Writing prompts can be a great way to begin generating ideas about your topic. For example, Berke (1995, pp. 89–90) suggested 20 questions that writers can use to develop their topics further. Even if you do not answer each of the questions, exploring even a few of these can help nudge you to that next level of understanding about your topic. We think the following ques-tions can be explored alone and on paper; however, we also believe talking through some of these questions with another person or small group can help you not only clarify the connection of these questions to your topic but also provide instant feedback as you generate your ideas for academic writing:

1. "How can X be described?"
2. "How did X happen?"
3. "What kind of person is X?"
4. "What is my memory of X?"
5. "What is my personal response to X?"
6. "What are the facts about X?"
7. "How can X be summarized?"
8. "What does X mean?"
9. "What is the essential function of X?"
10. "What are the component parts of X?"
11. "How is X made or done?"
12. "How should X be made or done?"
13. "What are the causes of X?"
14. "What are the consequences of X?"
15. "What are the types of X?"
16. "How does X compare to Y?"
17. "What is the present status of X?"
18. "How should X be interpreted?"
19. "What is the value of X?"
20. "What case can be made for or against X?"

Another use of writing prompts that Cowan and Cowan (1980, pp. 21–22) suggests to explore your topic is "cubing." Cubing entails taking your idea and imagining this idea as a cube. If you have ever held a Rubik's cube, you have the idea in your head of what the solid color sides of the cube look like. Then ask the following questions:

- Describe the topic—what is it?
- Compare it—what is it like or unlike?
- Associate it—what does it make you think of?
- Analyze it—what constituent parts is it made of?
- Apply it—how can it be used?
- Argue for and/or against it—how can you support or oppose it?

Again, responding to these questions alone and in writing is good, and talking through these questions as you "cube" your topic can generate even more information about your idea. Writing prompts can also be simple sentence stems like the following—kind of like fill-in-the-blank:

- "This topic is important because _____."
- "The important components of this topic are _____."
- "The part of this topic I am most interested in is _____."
- "When I am finished writing about this topic, I want to have said _____."

You get the idea. You can use these sentence stems, morph Berke's 20 questions and the cubing questions into sentence stems, or design your own sentence stems entirely.

Mind Maps

Another method of brainstorming that we like to use in idea generation is mind maps. Mind maps take all the stuff in your head about an idea that is jumbled up and maps it out into a visual depiction of the potential connections among the smaller portions of the idea you are exploring. We think mind maps not only help reveal these potential connections but also can be used in every type and stage of writing—from outlining an academic paper or identifying literature bases to explore to refining your dissertation topic. Figure 3.1 is an example of a mind map from a study Anneliese did on psychotherapy experiences of women of color survivors of child maltreatment.

In the mind map shown in Figure 3.1, you can see that Anneliese placed the topic—women of color survivors of child maltreatment—right in the center of the page. Then she began brainstorming potential connections

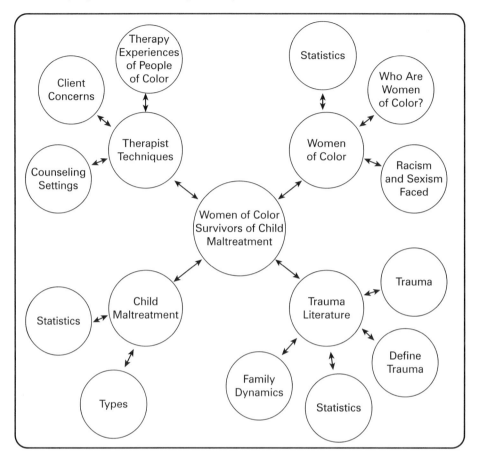

FIGURE 3.1. Mind mapping potential connections. From Hays and Singh (2012, p. 122). Copyright © 2012 The Guilford Press. Reprinted by permission.

from this central topic to other subtopics and their potential relationships. For instance, as Anneliese began to draw the connection to a subtopic of women of color, she immediately saw that she would need to discuss some statistics related to women of color as a group, as well as describing who this group is and exploring their experiences of racism and sexism.

Her mind map was a pretty simple exercise in getting the words and potential relationships on paper. However, you can get even more fancy and creative with mind maps. Buzan (n.d.) has provided a few suggestions on how to make a successful mind map and further unlock potential ideas:

1. Start in the center of a blank page turned sideways.
2. Use an image or picture for your central idea.
3. Use colors throughout.

4. Connect your main branches to the central image and connect your second- and third-level branches to the first and second levels and so forth.

5. Use images throughout.

Venn Diagrams

Once you have done some initial brainstorming using writing prompts and mind maps, creating Venn diagrams is a helpful way to deepen this exploration of your topic. Venn diagrams place topics within a series of circles in order to identify overlapping information among them. Just for your own information, you may hear both mind maps and Venn diagrams described as graphic organizers. Figure 3.2 shows a Venn diagram used to further generate ideas about the topic of career, leisure, and conflict among women:

Now, try your hand at using any of the techniques we have described to work with your own ideas for writing in Practice Exercise 3.4.

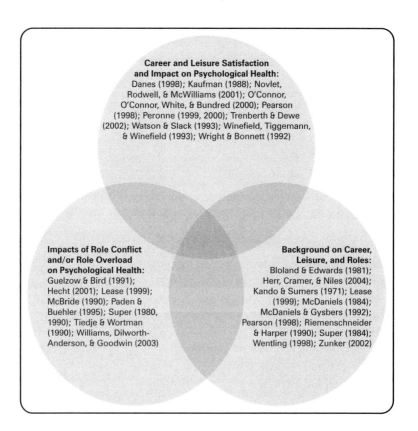

FIGURE 3.2. Venn diagram for generating ideas.

PRACTICE EXERCISE 3.4. Writing to Learn

- Select a topic in your discipline that appeals to you and one of the writing-to-learn techniques we described. Set a timer for 10 minutes. Use the technique you have chosen to explore the topic. Work quickly and don't let yourself get stuck thinking about any one thing for too long.
- After 10 minutes, stop. Take a break and walk away from what you have done for a few minutes. When you return, review what you have done and answer the following questions:
  1. What did you learn through your writing?
  2. Did you discover any connections or ideas that you hadn't thought of before?
  3. Do you want to continue adding ideas to what you have done? If yes, do so.

Writing Style

The strategies we have discussed thus far for finding your voice are predominantly related to finding the "content" and "approach" parts of your voice. These strategies may also help you find the "style" part of your voice, but they are not focused on finding your style. Many academic writers are relatively unaware of their own style or how they developed it. When it comes to style, they are most concerned with following the collective norms of their discipline. They simply want to fit in and produce writing that is like that of other members of their discipline's CoP. Once they achieve a degree of acceptance for their writing, they will probably continue to write in exactly the same way for years. They tend to think of academic writing as a formula, and once they believe that they have mastered the formula, they simply use that formula over and over again. There is actually nothing wrong with this approach as long as it works for you. However, this approach can lead to a nondescript writing voice, which of course decreases your chances of being unique in your discipline.

We suggest that newcomers may experience greater satisfaction with their own writing voices if they put more thought and intention into understanding and developing their writing styles. Academic writing is formulaic in many ways, but, as we illustrated earlier in this chapter, there are a variety of valid ways to achieve the formula. We suggest that newcomers understand that academic writing is made up of moves. *Moves* are things writers do to achieve specific writing goals. There are moves writers use for accomplishing more general goals, such as writing an introduction. For example, Swales (1990) is well known for his three-move model for introductions. In his model, which is widely accepted, to achieve the goals of an introduction to research writing, writers must (1) establish a research territory, (2) establish a niche or gap in that territory, and (3) occupy the niche or gap. Read through the excerpt from Kim (2014) and the commentary that accompanies it in Table 3.1 for a better understanding of the three-move model.

In academic writing, there are general moves any writer must achieve. Writing style is related to how individual writers achieve those general moves. As we discussed earlier, syntax, word choice, grammar choices, and punctuation can distinguish one writer from another in terms of how they achieve general moves in their writing. There are many ways to achieve the same move, but some are more common and more preferred in certain disciplines than others. The first step for newcomers is to learn the general moves. Learning the general moves can be the unconscious by-product of reading the same kinds of texts (e.g., experimental research articles) over and over. However, engaging in a more conscious process of analyzing the general moves can lead to a swifter understanding of the writing norms in your discipline. In fact, any time your professor gives you a model of a type of text that he would like you to write, your first step should be to analyze the moves of that text so that you have a clear understanding of what your professor expects.

Figuring out the general moves of texts in your field requires you to understand that academic writing has three structural levels. It has a macro-level structure, which we discussed in Chapter 1. This is the level at which texts such as research articles are divided into discrete sections. It also has a meso-level structure. This is the level at which sections are divided into paragraphs. Finally, it has a micro-level structure. This is the level at which sentences are grouped to form paragraphs and ideas are grouped to form sentences. The area of general moves is primarily related to the macro-level and meso-level of texts. The process for figuring out the moves of texts in your field is really quite easy if you just do the following:

- Divide the text into its macro-sections. This may be done for you if it is a research article that is already divided into sections.
- As you read each section, ask yourself, "What is the purpose of this section? What is the writer trying to accomplish in this section?" Don't get bogged down in details. Think about what the writer wants to accomplish in an overall sense for each section.
- Once you have an idea about the purpose of each section, read one section at a time. Ask yourself, "What moves did the writer make to achieve the purpose of this section?" Some sections may only have one move, but some may have many. Again, do not let yourself be distracted by the details of what the text says. Focus instead on what the writer does to achieve the purpose of the section.
- Find another text that is similar to the one you just analyzed (i.e., if you were working with an experimental article, find another

TABLE 3.1. Move Model for Introductions

Text

[1]The decision to attend college is a complex process. [2]It involves not only the college aspirants themselves, who prepare for, apply to, and choose a college, but also parents, families, communities, and school personnel. [3]Research has shown that parental involvement and socioeconomic status (SES) exert a significant influence on students' educational aspirations and college admission processes (Cabrera & La Nasa, 2000; Hossler, Schmit, & Vesper, 1999; Perna, 2000; Perna & Titus, 2005; Rowan-Kenyon, Bell, & Perna, 2008). [4]This influence may be complicated in a variety of ways. [5]Financial, psychological, and structural barriers often limit working-class or low-income parents' involvement in their children's transition to college, while high SES parents are able to provide information about and resources on the process of navigating college admission through various means, such as private counseling and tutoring to prepare for college entrance exams (e.g., Buchmann, Condron, & Roscingo, 2010; Deil-Amen & Tevis, 2010; Hoover-Dempsey & Sandler, 1997; Louie, 2001). [6]For example, Louie's (2001) study found marked differences between middle- and working-class Chinese immigrant parents in the allocation of educational resources to facilitate opportunities for a college education and social mobility for their children, calling for additional research on the impact of social class on parental educational strategies, access to college information and transmission of knowledge about the college application process.

[7]Parental involvement can also be complicated by race/ethnicity (Perna, 2000; Perna & Titus, 2005). [8]Perna and Titus have suggested that greater contact between parents and schools concerning academic issues is more likely to increase African American students' chances of enrolling in a four-year institution than it is for White, Hispanic, and Asian American students. [9]Teranishi, Ceja, Antonio, Allen, and McDonough (2004) found that both Chinese and Korean Americans were most likely to attend highly selective institutions, compared with other Asian ethnic groups (Filipino, Japanese, and Southeast Asian Americans). [10]Students from high-income backgrounds in these groups were also the most likely to take SAT preparation courses; more surprisingly, the rates of college prep course attendance for low-income Korean Americans were notably higher than those for other Asian ethnic groups, suggesting variation in the impact of both socioeconomic status and ethnicity on postsecondary preparation, opportunities, and decisions among Asian ethnic groups.

[11]While there is a growing body of research on the educational experiences and college choice process of ethnic groups in the Asian American population (Nakanishi, 1995; Park, 2012; Sue & Okazki, 1990; Takagi, 1992; Teranishi et al., 2004), scant attention has been paid, in particular, to how socioeconomic backgrounds affect the involvement of Asian immigrant parents in their children's postsecondary decisions and, conversely, how immigrant children negotiate their parents' expectations and involvement.

Commentary

Sentences 1–3 establish the research territory. The author orients the reader to the topics that will be discussed—the role of parental involvement and socioeconomic status in the decision-making and admission process of college-bound students. Sentences 4–10 establish the niche or gap in the research territory that the authors will address. In this case, the author establishes

(continued)

TABLE 3.1. *(continued)*

that there are a variety of impacts related to parental involvement and socioeconomic status and that these impacts affect the decision-making and admission process of different groups of college-bound youth in distinct ways. That is, they establish that impacts may vary across ethnic groups and within ethnic groups. In sentence 11, the author moves toward occupying the research niche by declaring her intentions to look specifically at the effect that socioeconomic backgrounds have on the involvement of Asian immigrant parents in their children's decision making. The author occupies the niche by narrowing her focus to a specific variable, socioeconomic status, and a specific group of parents, Asian immigrant parents, claiming that this combination has received less attention than other combinations.

experimental article). Repeat the process with this article and others. After only a few articles, you will realize that the moves of each article are fairly standard.

Once you have a firm grasp on the standard moves for texts in your discipline, you can move forward with investigating the style possibilities available to you. Style is not completely, but is mostly, a micro-level consideration. Earlier in this chapter, in Practice Exercise 3.1, we asked you to compare the style of two paragraphs at the micro-level. We provided our own commentary on this comparison in the Appendix. The benefit of looking at writing at the micro-level, especially of looking for micro-level patterns as we did in our commentary for Practice Exercise 3.1, is that you can find patterns that you can try out in your own writing. For example, you know that two standard moves of academic research writing are to establish a research niche or gap and to occupy it. In Table 3.1, Kim (2014) made the transition between establishing the gap and filling it with the following sentence:

> While there is a growing body of research on the educational experiences and college choice process of ethnic groups in the Asian American population (Nakanishi, 1995; Park, 2012; Sue & Okazki, 1990; Takagi, 1992; Teranishi et al., 2004), scant attention has been paid, in particular, to how socioeconomic backgrounds affect the involvement of Asian immigrant parents in their children's postsecondary decisions and, conversely, how immigrant children negotiate their parents' expectations and involvement.

If we break this sentence down on a micro-level, we can see the pattern the author used to achieve this move. She began with a contrast signaled by the introductory clause beginning with *while*. She followed the introductory clause with the term *scant*, which indicates absence or lack. After indicating the existence of an absence or gap, she specified what was missing, and these missing topics are understood as her own research focus. The pattern is something like the following:

- State what research does exist (must contrast with what you intend to study).
- State that something is missing from that research.
- Specify what is missing from that research (must be the topics that you investigated).

Obviously, this pattern can be used to write about many topics, and it can be varied in many ways. We could replace *while* with *although*. We could replace *scant attention* with *little research*. And, of course, we can replace the content of the sentence with any content.

You already know that every research article you read is going to have moves such as establishing the gap and occupying the gap. Once you know this, you can simply pay attention to the variety of ways in which each author chooses to accomplish this move on a micro-level. You will find that some authors' choices appeal to you more than others, and we encourage you to follow their patterns. Now, to be clear, we are not encouraging you to plagiarize. We are encouraging you to emulate more experienced writers. We fully expect that you can and will use your own words and ideas to follow their patterns. See Box 3.1 for Lauren's story of emulating writers and then innovating her own writing.

INTEGRATING YOUR VOICE WITH OTHERS' VOICES

One of the key aspects of developing your own writing voice entails knowing how voice is typically used in academic writing. Typically, writing scholars have identified two components: *indirect voice* and *direct voice*. Direct voice refers to the use of your own voice or other scholars' voices. For instance, direct voice might include your own ideas or direct quotes from other scholars. Indirect voice refers to paraphrasing another scholar's ideas or summarizing a group of scholars' ideas.

In terms of your direct voice, we began to talk about the idea of your own academic writing voice in Chapter 1, and this discussion continues throughout each chapter of the book. As we have discussed, there are a variety of ways to express your own academic writing voice. However, things get a bit tricky when using the direct voice of others. First and foremost, you must cite direct quotations to avoid plagiarism. This is a major issue of ethics and integrity within academic writing and scholarship in general. Second, depending upon the field you are in, direct voice may be used a lot, a little, or not very much at all. For instance, in peer-reviewed journal articles in education, the use of long direct quotes from scholars is pretty common. See how Hwahng and Nuttbrock (2014, p. 693) use a direct quote when discussing transgender women of color in New York City:

Another focus was on "intersectional perspective," in which simultaneous dimensions of inequality are examined, including how these dimensions are interrelated and how they shape and influence one another.

> Understanding the racial and ethnic experiences of sexual- and gender-minority individuals requires taking into account the full range of *historical* and *social experiences* both within and between sexual- and gender-minority groups with respect to class, gender, race, ethnicity, and geographical location. (IOM, 2011, p. 21, italics added)

However, in Anneliese's field of counseling and psychology, the use of direct quotes is pretty minimal. Therefore, if she is selecting a direct quote from another scholar, for instance, about women of color survivors of child maltreatment, she wants to make sure she cannot put this author's words into a paraphrase or summary; essentially, the use of direct quotes is called for when the original author shares her idea in a way that is salient, powerful, and not as easy to put in other words.

BOX 3.1. Emulating and Innovating

When I was in college, I had the opportunity to study abroad in Madrid one summer. I was particularly impressed by the art museum El Prado, and I visited it more than once. While I was there, I noticed multiple artists with their easels and paints set up who appeared to be copying the renowned art works displayed. I really couldn't see why anyone would want to copy another person's work day after day. It made no sense to my young self. I did not see how it would improve the work of artists who spent all of their time copying the work of others. Much later in life, I realized the importance of the process that I had witnessed. Yes, these artists were copying others' work, but as they copied, they learned techniques and developed skills that they may not have had before. They were required to do things as they copied that they had perhaps never attempted in their original works of art. Of course, these techniques and skills could then be applied in their original art. In addition, I imagine that in the process of copying another's work, an artist may experience the desire to improve upon the original with some new idea that has occurred to him. In these moments, the artist is experiencing the integration of his own experiences with those of the master, and the result is something new and unique. I see developing your own writing voice, especially with regard to style, in much the same way. You must first mimic others who are further along than you, but as your understanding of what they are doing deepens, you will acquire techniques and discover stylistic innovations that belong to you.

—Lauren

For example, Anneliese found the way that the following idea was expressed to be salient and powerful:

> Child maltreatment is a formidable problem in the United States. (Patel et al., 2012, p. 2)

So, she might use a section of this quote and embed a smaller section of the quote in her own writing to provide more emphasis on her topic in the following manner:

> Scholars have asserted that child maltreatment is a "formidable problem in the United States" (Patel et al., 2012, p. 2), with rates of child maltreatment escalating over the past decade.

A large part of your own direct voice as an academic writer is being able to use direct quotes in alignment with the way they are typically used in your discipline *and* continuing to develop your own direct voice. Talking with advanced students in your discipline about how they developed a strong academic writing voice can give you some insight into the emotional components of this process and provide you with some easy-to-implement wisdom. Take a look at what counselor education doctoral student Brandee Appling says about developing her writing voice:

> "As a first year doctoral student I remember struggling with conceptualizing academic writing. After submitting my first paper in my doctoral program, I was told that I needed to work on finding my voice. I remember feeling perplexed about what my professor meant when she said that my voice was not showing up in my writing. I struggled with identifying my academic writing voice. I was confident in my writing abilities so I knew it was there but I just could not find it. The first year of my doctoral program I tried to write something 'academic' everyday, even if it was just for a few minutes. I had to push aside my inhibitions and self-doubt, and just start writing. The more I wrote, the more I began to notice that my writing had a distinct style that was uniquely mine. In addition to writing every day, I began to speak the language. I would often read my own writing or the writing of others out loud, so that I hear the nuances and feel the flow of the words. I began to familiarize myself with new terms and phrases in my discipline. Then, I would incorporate these into my everyday conversation in order to become comfortable with using academic, formal writing terms. Finding my academic voice has been like learning a new language. It was, and still is, a growing process that I continue to refine."

As Brandee shared, strengthening your voice entails getting familiar with what you know and what you are not yet as familiar with in your discipline. This brings us right back to one of the foundations of good writing—curiosity—in which you are thinking about, reflecting on, and analyzing your writing.

CHAPTER SUMMARY AND REMINDERS

In this chapter, we have defined academic writing voice as a pattern of choices that distinguishes you from other writers in your discipline. Content, approach, and style are all choices that contribute to finding your academic voice. The process of making these choices begins early in your graduate career and continues well beyond your graduation. We have described several actions you can take as you participate in this process that we believe will help you enjoy this process and get the most out of it. See Summary Table 3.1 for awareness and action reminders.

SUMMARY TABLE 3.1. AWARENESS AND ACTION REMINDERS	
Be aware . . .	Take action . . .
Norms are not etched in concrete—they are malleable.	Look for inspirational voices in the texts you read.
Academic writing voice is a reflection of the choices that writers make regarding content, approach, and expression.	Invite your personal curiosity to be part of your academic voice.
Academic writers must fit in and stand out—that is, they must communicate with the collective voice and their own unique voice.	Use writing as a way to discover your voice.
Academic writing is a series of strategic but predictable moves.	Emulate other writers to innovate your own style.

UNIT II
DEVELOPING ACADEMIC WRITING SKILLS

CHAPTER 4

Understanding Academic Writer–Reader Roles and Writing Structures

As we have previously discussed, newcomers to the academic writing CoP have to learn how to communicate like full members. This means that they have to learn academic writing language. However, learning academic writing language is something more than just learning new words or a new style of expression. Language is an external expression, but it is also a reflection of how people think—not just their opinions or ideas but their actual thought patterns. Thus newcomers to the academic writing CoP really need to learn how to think like full members as part of learning to use academic writing language.

In this chapter, our **awareness focus** is on helping you to gain a deeper understanding of how the structure of academic writing language is specifically related to writer–reader roles. Our **action focus** includes ideas for steps that you can take to increase your familiarity with the thought patterns underlying the language and to develop your ability to use them.

WRITER–READER ROLES

When people communicate with one another, they rely to a large extent on their personal familiarity with one another, whether that means knowing how the other thinks or knowing which words and phrases will be understood the best. For example, when teachers communicate with students in their classrooms, they can use whatever shorthand they have established in their classes for discussing specific topics. The shorthand used by the teacher might not make sense to someone outside of the class, but that does not matter because the person receiving the communication understands it. When roles communicate with one another, there is no personal familiarity and no shorthand. So the chances of misunderstandings are much greater. Academic writing language creates a kind of artificial familiarity or shorthand between writers and readers that they can use to avoid misunderstandings. Writers and readers share a way of thinking and expressing themselves that allows writers to communicate with readers across space, time, and even different disciplines in ways that are understandable. Thus, learning how to think and communicate in academic writing language is the key to expressing your voice in academic writing.

One of the unusual things about academic writing language is that it is not a language that people usually speak. It is for the most part strictly a written language. And it is also for the most part a language that has developed for writers to communicate with readers rather than for people to communicate with one another. This may sound like a strange thing to say, but understanding that writers and readers are not the same as people is actually quite important for understanding how to think and communicate in academic writing language.

Writers and readers hold distinctly different roles in academic writing that go beyond just the obvious fact that one is writing and one is reading. In academic research writing, writers and readers are engaged in a kind of imaginary debate regarding the strength of the writer's argument. The writer's role is that of persuader. The writer is proposing a new idea or a new perspective on an existing idea, and is attempting to provide a sound, credible, and logical argument that the reader will accept as valid and reasonable. The point of persuasion in academic writing is not to literally persuade the reader to agree with you. The reader may not agree with you, but academic readers can be persuaded to see your point of view as worthy of consideration. As a graduate student, you often spend much more time in the reader role (e.g., critiquing articles you have read), whereas the time you spend in the writer role (e.g., writing one paper a semester) may be less—so spending more time in the writer role is important and takes practice.

The reader's role in these interactions is that of doubter. Readers approach academic texts from a critical perspective. Their job is to question everything from the writers' decisions to their methods to their interpretations. They look for conceptual flaws, inaccurate or misrepresented content, and stylistic errors that create confusion and/or diminish credibility. They evaluate every aspect of a written text in terms of how it either strengthens or weakens the writer's argument. Obviously, writers do not necessarily know how readers evaluate their texts unless they have formally submitted them for evaluation, for instance to a professor or to a journal. Regardless, the very fact that readers are questioning and evaluating written texts creates one of the most notable essential characteristics of academic writing—audience awareness.

AUDIENCE AWARENESS

Audience awareness refers to the general idea that speakers and writers must be very attuned to and aware of their intended or imagined audiences when they speak or write. Audience awareness in academic writing is heightened. That is, academic writers have a high conscious, as well as unconscious, level of awareness of their audience's expectations. This high level of awareness is a prominent thought pattern in academic writing that influences writers' communication with their audience and is responsible for many of the essential characteristics of academic writing language.

Of course, the audience for academic writing comprises the readers, who, as we already explained, are not people but roles. In academic writing, writers generally attend simultaneously to two audiences or types of readers. One audience or reader is the imaginary general academic audience, the doubting reader that we have already described. The other audience or reader is the intended audience, which is also an imaginary audience but is one that is specifically chosen by the writer. All academic writing must have a raison d'être. It must have a justification for being that responds to the proverbial "So what?" and "Who cares?" questions. The writer's intended audience is typically related to both the writer's topic and the manner in which she intends to answer the "Who cares?" question. Just as considerations about the imagined doubting reader affect writers' decisions about how to express themselves using academic writing language, so too do considerations about the intended audience's knowledge of the writer's topic, their feelings about the topic, and the value they put on the topic. The overarching impact of all of these considerations on academic writing language has been the development of an extremely writer-responsible approach to writing.

WRITER-RESPONSIBLE WRITING

Hinds (1987) used the terms *writer-responsible* and *reader-responsible* to describe the degree to which different cultures expect the writer or the reader, respectively, to make sense of a written text. Writer-responsible cultures expect the writer to explain everything very clearly to the reader, whereas reader-responsible cultures expect readers to bring more to the table and to do more work in making sense of a text. His view has been criticized as overgeneralizing when it comes to discussions of other languages and cultures, but it does provide a useful point of view for understanding the relationship between the writer and the reader. For example, we can apply Hinds's view to different types of writing, such as poetry versus recipes. Poetry uses language in figurative ways to express emotions and thoughts in an artistic manner. Writers and readers of poetry expect readers to figure out what it means, and it is perfectly acceptable for different readers to come up with different meanings. Therefore, poetry is more reader-responsible. In contrast, recipes are writer-responsible. Both writers and readers of recipes know that the writer is supposed to write in a step-by-step, clear manner that will allow the reader to physically follow the writer's directions. Every step in the process is spelled out so that readers do not have to interpret or guess the meaning.

According to Hinds's model, U.S. academic writing tends to be strongly writer-responsible. This means that the basic expectation of U.S. writing is that the writer will assume almost complete responsibility for making sure that his written message is clearly explained to the reader. The writer will seek to avoid any confusion by carefully organizing his ideas and providing definitions, explanations, and examples. The writer will not expect the reader to figure out how ideas are related to one another. Rather, the writer will attempt to anticipate and appropriately address any aspect of his writing that might lead to even momentary confusion on the part of the reader. And, importantly, the reader *expects* the writer to do all of this.

In writer-responsible writing, the writer's heightened audience awareness allows and requires her to imagine how readers will respond to her text before the readers even see it. This ability to imagine responses in turn allows and requires writers to take specific steps to circumvent or mitigate possible negative responses while courting positive responses, and again all of this happens before readers even see the text. All of this imagined interaction between writer and reader roles is a cultural thought pattern that precedes actual writing. When thoughts are actually transferred into writing, this thought pattern of anticipating and responding to readers is manifested in one of the essential characteristics of academic writing, which is academic writers' use of coherent structure.

COHERENT STRUCTURE

In writing, structure refers to the organization of ideas in a text. It is the order in which the ideas are presented. The structure of a text is its framework. The framework helps writers and readers to know where specific ideas should be presented. Different types of texts require different structures because they reflect different ideas about how writers and readers think. For example, newspaper articles are often written using an inverted pyramid structure wherein the most important information is given at the beginning and the information that follows is presented in decreasing order of importance. Writers and readers of newspapers share a way of thinking that prioritizes delivering the basic *who, what, when, where, why,* and *how* facts as soon as possible. Thus the structure reflects their shared understanding and makes it easy for them to understand one another.

In academic writing, a coherent structure is preferred. Coherent means logical, clear, and orderly. In writer-responsible writing, the use of a coherent structure makes the reader's job easier and decreases the possibility of misunderstandings. The concept of coherence can be a bit tricky in the writer–reader relationship, because, of course, it is always possible that the writer and the reader have different ideas as to what is a logical, clear, and orderly structure. This is often the case when newcomers are writing for full members. However, in academic writing, it is the writer's job to write for the reader's sense of coherence rather than his own, meaning that the writer needs to think like the reader so that he can anticipate and fix any structural issues that may cause confusion for the reader. In other words, the writer has to know very well how the reader reads, and in academic writing, the reader reads with specific structural expectations.

Reading is all about expectations. When we read, we are constantly formulating expectations and making predictions, consciously and unconsciously. When we come to a point in our reading where something does not match our expectations or predictions, we feel confused. We may reread something at that point to try to figure out the problem. However, if we reread and find that the problem is not our reading comprehension but the writer's lack of coherence, we feel annoyed and frustrated.

In writer-responsible writing, the writer's goal is to *not* annoy the readers by confusing them. In fact, in academic writing, the writer is trying to match her thought pattern to that of the reader, which sounds really improbable when you consider all of the possible readers that a text could have. However, remember that writers and readers who both use academic writing language have similar thought and expression patterns by virtue of knowing how to use the language, so they have or should have similar ideas of what coherent structure is.

In academic writing, coherent structure is something that writers must use and create on multiple levels. We think of these levels as the macro-, meso-, and micro-levels of writing. The macro-level structure of academic writing is the overall structure of the text. It includes the section and subsection titles (some may be predetermined by the text type, but others are decided by the writer). The macro-level reflects the general thought progression the writer believes the reader needs in order to accept the writer's argument. The meso-level is the organization of ideas within sections or subsections; you might think of this as the order of paragraphs within a section. The meso-level reflects the thought progression that the writer believes the reader needs to understand the main point of the section or subsection. The micro-level is the organization of sentences within a paragraph. It reflects the thought progression that the writer believes the reader needs to understand the point of the paragraph.

We would like to emphasize again that coherent structure is as much about how writers think as how they write, so any writing patterns they use are actually reflective of a pattern of thinking. As we have discussed in Chapters 1–3, academic writing in general uses a problematizing approach, so the overarching thought pattern is for the writer to identify a problem and lead the reader to a logical "solution" (i.e., problem–solution pattern). In this case, solution does not mean that the problem was actually solved. In fact, it would be more accurate to say that the writer leads the reader to a new or at least updated conclusion with regard to the problem (i.e., problem–conclusion pattern). The conclusion is not actually likely to be a "solution" in the common sense of the word; it is more likely to be the suggestion that the reader adopt a new or expanded perspective. If the argument is coherent, the reader is more likely to be persuaded to consider the writer's point of view about the problem. To that end, academic research writing requires the writer to include certain standard steps in the overarching problem–conclusion pattern.

For example, writers must identify and problematize gaps. They must situate those gaps in relation to past research, and they must propose unique ways to address those gaps through their research. They must explain how they did their research and share data resulting from their research. They must explain what their data mean and how they help to address the gaps that the writers have identified. They must acknowledge limitations in their research and propose future directions for research that would expand upon their findings.

Within the overarching problem–conclusion pattern, inside of the previously mentioned steps, writers structure and express their thoughts using a variety of other patterns. Because writers are trying to persuade readers to see a problem the way that the writers themselves see it, they choose organizational patterns by considering what pattern would be the clearest and easiest for readers to follow. Writers know that if readers find something easy to follow, they will likely evaluate the argument as following a coherent structure. There are four particular organization patterns that can be found in most academic research writing: hierarchical organization, classification, cause–effect organization, and parallelism. Thus these are some of the most important patterns for new writers to understand and use.

Hierarchical Organizational Pattern

As a disclaimer, the name that we have given to this pattern is *not* official writing terminology. However, we feel that the hierarchical descriptor allows us to talk about a few ways of organizing that are quite similar. This pattern of thinking and expression involves beginning with a concept that is "more" or "bigger" in some way and moving to something that is "less" or "smaller." Writers use this pattern when their ideas are not all equal in some way. For example, they could be unequal because one idea is more important, or they could be unequal because one idea is more general than another.

This particular pattern is probably so common in academic writing because it basically reflects the thought progression of argumentation. To argue something, writers must begin with a bigger point and support it with more detailed evidence. To evaluate an argument, readers want to know where to find the biggest or most important point so that they can assess the relevance and quality of the evidence. The hierarchical pattern helps both writer and reader roles to organize their respective tasks. Writers express their thoughts using the hierarchical pattern as much as possible at all three structural levels.

Macro-Level

At the macro-level, sections (if not predetermined by the article type) will typically be organized insofar as possible in a hierarchical pattern. Subsections, which are almost always determined by the writer, will also be organized in this way. For example, Bugg (2013) analyzed the controversy over the building of a Hindu temple in Sydney, Australia. She used this controversy to illustrate how citizenship does not necessarily guarantee migrant religious groups the same rights or treatment as other citizens. Her article included some predetermined sections, but she also determined many of the sections. Review her sections and the commentary that accompanies them in Table 4.1 to see how a hierarchical pattern is applied at the macro-level.

TABLE 4.1. Hierarchical Organization at the Macro-Level

Macro-level sections

  I. Introduction

  II. Citizenship, Belonging and Landscape

  III. Citizenship and Belonging in the Australian Context

  IV. The Rural–Urban Fringe, Citizenship and Belonging

  V. Context and Methodology

  VI. Citizenship and Belonging in the Hindu Temple Case Study

  VII. Conclusions

Commentary

Sections I, V, and VII would fall into the category of predetermined categories, so we will exclude them from consideration. The remaining sections follow a clear hierarchical organization. Section II introduces the reader to the more general concepts of citizenship, belonging, and landscape. Section III retakes those same topics but introduces the reader to those concepts in a more specific way by limiting the discussion to the Australian context. Section IV continues with the topics but introduces the reader to an even more specific context, the rural–urban fringe (of Australian cities), and, finally, section VI moves the discussion to a very specific example—a case study. As you can see just from the section titles, the ideas of each section are related to one another, but they are unequal in the sense that some ideas are "bigger" in scope than others. Thus the hierarchical organization helps writers communicate how their thoughts are moving from one level to another, becoming increasingly more specific.

Meso-Level

Writers can also use a hierarchical approach at the meso-level. For example, they may discuss the idea they consider to be the most salient in the first paragraph and the ideas they consider to be less salient in the second and third paragraphs. Or they may discuss the idea that is bigger in the sense that more research has been done on it in the first paragraph and the ideas that are smaller in the sense that there is less research in the following paragraphs. The hierarchical organization at the meso-level is quite noticeable in introductions because the thought progression of an introduction is usually from a bigger general topic to a smaller, more specific subtopic to the focus of the study. For example, review the first sentence from each of the four paragraphs of Kuhlen, Galati, and Brennan (2012, pp. 18–19) in Box 4.1 and notice how the concepts addressed go from bigger to smaller (see the underlined words), moving from the bigger concept of conversation to the influence of top-down and bottom-up sources of information on gestures.

Micro-Level

The hierarchical pattern is most obvious at the micro-level. This pattern may be the framework for a whole paragraph, or it may be a pattern that repeats itself within a single paragraph. See the first paragraph of Choi and Miller's (2014, p. 340) literature review and the commentary that accompanies it in Table 4.2, explaining how they use a hierarchical structure.

BOX 4.1. Hierarchical Organization at the Meso-Level

1. Conversation involves coordination, not only *intra*personally, but also *inter*personally.

2. Both verbal and nonverbal signals are smoothly integrated into utterances, and yet the two kinds of signals seem quite different.

3. As speakers adapt the verbal and nonverbal aspects of their utterances to their addressees, they can draw from: (a) top-down information such as expectations about their addressees, and (b) bottom-up information that unfolds during the interaction, such as feedback that signals addressees' engagement, uptake, understanding, and informational needs as the conversation unfolds.

4. In this paper, we examine how top-down and bottom-up sources of information each contribute to how speakers gesture during spontaneous narrative, and how such factors may influence one another.

TABLE 4.2. Hierarchical Organization at the Micro-Level
Micro-level (paragraph)
[1]According to Corrigan (2004), stigma is one of the most common reasons that individuals are unwilling to seek counseling. [2]*Stigma toward counseling* refers to an individual's perception of the devaluation, rejection, and discrimination that may occur if the individual receives counseling (Major & O'Brien, 2005; Yang et al., 2007). [3]Stigma toward counseling is related to less positive attitudes toward seeking professional help and a diminished willingness to seek counseling (Ludwikowski et al., 2009; Vogel et al., 2006; 2007). [4]Stigma toward counseling is an especially relevant construct for AAPI populations, who tend to report higher levels of stigma toward seeking counseling than other cultural groups (Gilbert et al., 2007). [5]Studies have shown negative relationships between stigma and attitudes toward seeking counseling and between stigma and mental health service utilization among AAPI individuals (Eisenberg, Downs, Golberstein, & Zivin, 2009; Kandula, Kersey, & Lurie, 2004; Shea & Yeh, 2008).
Commentary
Sentence 1 introduces the authors' general claim of the existence of *stigma* being related to unwillingness to seek counseling. In this case, the authors' claim is actually the claim of an outside source. Nonetheless, as the authors are the ones making the argument in this particular paragraph, it is now also *their* claim. In other words, they have aligned themselves with this claim. Sentence 2 reduces the topic of the claim slightly to *stigma toward counseling* and provides a *general definition* of this reduced topic. It also cites other sources to support the credibility of their definition. Sentence 3 reduces stigma toward counseling a bit more by focusing on how it relates to *less positive attitudes toward seeking counseling* and cites sources to provide credible evidence that the relationship the authors claim really exists. Sentence 4 reduces the topic of seeking counseling to a specific group, *AAPI populations*, and cites a source to provide credible evidence that this relationship really exists. Sentence 5 reduces to providing *detailed credible evidence* that AAPI populations do indeed have a stigma toward seeking counseling.
As you can see, the point of the paragraph was to lead readers through a thought process that would allow them to follow the authors' reasoning and provide proof that the authors followed a logical line of reasoning—it's very similar to the idea of "showing your work" when you do a math problem. The reader wants to know how the writer arrived at any claim so that the reader can evaluate the strength of the claim.

In the case of Table 4.2, the authors had to think like readers and anticipate the following:

- Readers need to know our general claim. They must be oriented to our general topic.
    - What are we trying to argue in this paragraph in the most general sense?
    - Is our general claim supported by other credible sources?

- Readers need to know how we define the terms of our claim. If readers understand the terms differently than we do, they will not be able to follow our reasoning.
  - ○ What is our working definition of terms involved in our claim?
  - ○ Is our working definition supported by other credible sources?
- Readers need to know how we are reducing our general claim to something more specific.
  - ○ Where are we trying to go with our general claim in more specific terms?
  - ○ Is there credible evidence to support going in this direction?
- Readers need to know the exact parameters within which we are situating our claim.
  - ○ What exactly are we arguing in its most specific terms?
  - ○ Is our very specific claim supported by other credible sources?
- Readers need to know that we have done our due diligence as academic writers and found evidence that has empirically indicated the validity of our claim.
  - ○ What evidence have we found that supports the validity of our claim?

The most important advice that we would give any writer trying to create and express a coherent structure is to ask yourself, "What does my reader need to know now?" at each point in your writing. This is true regardless of the pattern you choose to use. Asking yourself about the reader shifts the focus from you writing for yourself to you writing for someone who does not know what you know. This shift is extremely important, as writers tend to produce reader-responsible rather than writer-responsible writing when they write for themselves. Try to work through Bugg's (2013, p. 1153) thought process as we did in our commentary on Table 4.2 by completing Practice Exercise 4.1. You can check your answers in the Appendix.

PRACTICE EXERCISE 4.1. Anticipating the Reader's Expectations

Read the excerpt and answer the accompanying questions.

TEXT

[1]As noted above, most of the recent conflicts around planning for minority religious spaces have taken place in the rural–urban fringe of Australia's metropolitan areas. [2]In using the term "rural–urban fringe" I refer to the zone of transition along the urban–rural continuum. [3]I use the word "continuum"

to indicate the lack of jarring shifts or line of demarcation between urban and rural. [4]While there is significant literature on rural–urban linkages or the "peri-urban fringe" (see Simon, 2008 for a review), my work focuses on the discourse of the rural as incubator of certain cultural values, and the implications of a shifting demography for those cultural values. [5]With Cloke, I note the significance of the social construction of the rural, even in the face of the absence of a functioning "rural." [6]As he states, although "the *geographical* spaces of urban and rural are being broken down, the imagined opposition between the social significance of urban and rural are being maintained and in some ways enhanced" (Cloke 2004:21; his italics). [7]Australian fringe areas are typically areas of significant population growth and are located in areas of high environmental value (Houston 2005). [8]As metropolitan areas rapidly encroach upon these rural fringe areas, there are greater demands on rural land, from "the provision of ecosystem services, amenities and aesthetics" to the "preservation of cultural landscapes" (McCarthy 2005:774).

COMMENTARY

1. What does the author think the reader needs to know in sentence 1? What question(s) is the author attempting to answer with sentence 1?
2. What does the author think the reader needs to know in sentence 2? What question(s) is the author attempting to answer with sentence 2?
3. What does the author think the reader needs to know in sentence 3? What question(s) is the author attempting to answer with sentence 3?
4. What does the author think the reader needs to know in sentence 4? What question(s) is the author attempting to answer with sentence 4?
5. What does the author think the reader needs to know in sentence 5? What question(s) is the author attempting to answer with sentence 5?
6. What does the author think the reader needs to know in sentence 6? What question(s) is the author attempting to answer with sentence 6?
7. What does the author think the reader needs to know in sentence 7? What question(s) is the author attempting to answer with sentence 7?
8. What does the author think the reader needs to know in sentence 8? What question(s) is the author attempting to answer with sentence 8?

The Language of Hierarchical Organization

As we have discussed, the hierarchical organization pattern is related to the order of ideas—from more to less or bigger to smaller—so, in many ways, what writers are doing is just narrowing down the beginning idea to ideas that are more and more specific. In doing so, writers utilize a few language strategies that can be helpful at any level but may be particularly helpful at the micro-level.

Word Choice

One language strategy that writers use is related to word choice. Words exist on a couple of different continua. One continuum is from abstract to concrete, and the other is from general to specific. The abstract-to-concrete continuum is related to the intangible versus the tangible qualities of words. Abstract words are intangible, and we understand them through our thoughts. Concrete words are tangible, and we understand them through actual physical experiences of them. For example, love is abstract, whereas a kiss is concrete. The general-to-specific continuum is related to broad categories versus individual instances. For example, animal is a very broad category, border collie is a narrower category, and Fido is a specific individual instance of the category.

Writers can use terms that are more abstract or general at the beginning of a hierarchical structure to discuss their claims in more general terms, and they can become increasingly more specific in their selection of terms as they approach the end. Consider how a writer could use the following words as he creates a coherent structure for an argument that is ultimately related to the importance of using iPads:

- Technology
- Personal computers
- Laptops
- Mobile devices
- Tablets
- iPads

Noun Phrases

Noun phrases are parts of sentences that function as nouns, usually subjects and objects. A noun phrase can begin with one word and be expanded to many through the addition of a variety of modifiers. In academic writing, beginning with simple noun phrases and expanding those noun phrases incrementally is another language strategy that writers use to express their claims in hierarchical terms. Consider how the expansion of the original noun phrase in the following list would support a hierarchical organizational pattern:

- Students
- International students
- Undergraduate international students
- Prematriculated undergraduate international students

- Prematriculated undergraduate international students who are seeking admission to U.S. colleges and universities
- Prematriculated undergraduate international students who are seeking admission to the top 25 engineering programs in U.S. colleges and universities

Signal Words or Phrases

Signal words or phrases are expressions that writers use to indicate the path that they are following. Because the writer is responsible for guiding the reader in academic writing, writers use signal words or phrases to help readers understand the organizational pattern they are using to express their thoughts. In a hierarchical pattern, writers use a wide array of signal words or phrases to indicate their movement from more to less or bigger to smaller. We also recommend that you simply Google "signal words" or "transition words" for more lists of words and phrases that you can use. We find the list at *www.smart-words.org/linking-words/transition-words.html* to be particularly helpful.

See Table 4.3 for a detailed commentary of how Choi and Miller (2014, p. 340) used language to present and support their claim using a hierarchical organizational pattern.

Classification

Classification is another common pattern for organizing and expressing thoughts in academic writing. When using the classification pattern, writers generally break a bigger topic down into smaller topics, which is similar to the hierarchical pattern. However, in the case of classification, the writer sees the smaller topics as different from one another but equal. In other words, the order in which the writer chooses to express the smaller topics is not based on principles of hierarchy.

This pattern of thought and expression is probably common in academic writing for two reasons. One reason is that academic writing is based on analysis, and analysis implies breaking things down into parts. Another reason is the fact that academic writing is extremely writer-responsible. The writer is responsible for the reader's understanding, so it makes sense that breaking larger topics into smaller topics would make the writer's task of explaining everything very clearly to the reader easier.

Like the hierarchical strategy, you can find evidence of classification at all levels of academic writing. For example, in Box 4.2, you can see that Singh and McKleroy (2011, p. 38) created subsections in their Findings section based on themes that they found. The order of the themes is not hierarchical, cause-and-effect, or chronological, because the themes are all equal.

TABLE 4.3. Language Use in Hierarchical Organizational Patterns

Text	Commentary
[1]According to Corrigan (2004), stigma is one of the most common reasons that individuals are unwilling to seek counseling.	• The use of "is one of the most common" indicates that the authors are beginning at the top of a hierarchy that includes many possibilities that are not equal to the one that they will discuss. • The use of "individuals" indicates that the authors are presenting information in very general terms, because it is such a general word.
[2]*Stigma toward counseling* refers to an individual's perception of the devaluation, rejection, and discrimination that may occur if the individual receives counseling (Major & O'Brien, 2005; Yang et al., 2007).	• The authors create an expanded noun phrase "stigma toward counseling" to narrow the subject introduced in the first sentence. • They use "refers to" to indicate that they will be narrowing the discussion by defining the terms of their claim.
[3]Stigma toward counseling is related to less positive attitudes toward seeking professional help and a diminished willingness to seek counseling (Ludwikowski et al., 2009; Vogel et al., 2006; 2007).	• The use of "is related to" indicates that the authors are narrowing their discussion further by introducing a specific relationship. • The authors use two expanded noun phrases, "less positive attitudes toward seeking professional help" and "a diminished willingness to seek counseling," to narrow and clarify what they mean by "unwilling to seek counseling," an idea they introduced in sentence 1 as part of their general claim.
[4]Stigma toward counseling is an especially relevant construct for AAPI populations, who tend to report higher levels of stigma toward seeking counseling than other cultural groups (Gilbert et al., 2007).	• The authors signal that the reader has reached their most specific claim with the noun phrase "especially relevant construct for AAPI populations." The reader understands that the subject, "stigma toward counseling" that was narrowed from just "stigma" in sentence 2 has now been narrowed to be something that is related to one very specific group. • The use of the specific term "AAPI populations" replaces the general term "individuals."
[5]Studies have shown negative relationships between stigma and attitudes toward seeking counseling and between stigma and mental health service utilization among AAPI individuals (Eisenberg, Downs, Golberstein, & Zivin, 2009; Kandula, Kersey, & Lurie, 2004; Shea & Yeh, 2008).	• "Studies have shown" indicates that the authors will now provide specific evidence of the previously stated claim. • The expanded noun phrases "attitudes toward seeking counseling" and "mental health service utilization" narrow the concept of "counseling" to more specific aspects of counseling.

> **BOX 4.2. Classification at the Macro-Level**
>
> There were six major themes common to all participants' experiences of resilience as transgender people of color who had survived traumatic life experiences: (a) pride in one's gender and ethnic/racial identity, (b) recognizing and negotiating gender and racial/ethnic oppression, (c) navigating relationships with family, (d) accessing health care and financial resources, (e) connecting with an activist transgender community of color, and (f) cultivating spirituality and hope for the future (see Figure 1).

The classification organizing pattern can also be found at the meso-level. At the meso-level, it would be most common in sections in which enumeration is not related to any particular relationship between the topics enumerated, as is the case in the Limitations and Future Directions for Research section of Choi and Miller (2014, p. 349). In Table 4.4 you can see a few sentences from each of the three paragraphs in the section. Notice how these few sentences indicate that a classification organizational pattern is being used that is not based on any particular connection between the topics.

TABLE 4.4. Classification at the Meso-Level

Paragraph 1
Present findings should be considered in light of a number of study limitations. First, there are sample-related limitations. Our convenience sample consisted of AAPI undergraduate and graduate students at a large mid-Atlantic university; therefore, the generalizability of findings across AAPI populations is unclear.
Paragraph 2
Another study limitation (which pervades AAPI psychological research) relates to the meaningfulness (or meaninglessness) of aggregating unique Asian and Pacific Islander ethnic groups into a unified AAPI population, even though there is diversity among these groups.
Paragraph 3
Although we focused on AAPI individuals' willingness to seek (professional) counseling, there are a number of other (perhaps more ecologically valid) sources of help for AAPI populations. For example, researchers have highlighted the ways in which Asian ethnic churches and extended family structures provide unique mental health support for AAPI populations (Choi, Yang, Huh, Hill, & Miller, 2013; Min & Kim, 2005). In future research, they can explore further the understanding of AAPI individuals' unique experiences related to seeking professional and nonprofessional help.

TABLE 4.5. Classification at the Micro-Level
Text
[1]There appear to be several potential relationships among the major themes in this study, such as the relationship between developing pride in one's racial/ethnic and gender identities and the themes of family support and/or connecting with a transgender people of color community. [2]Future research could examine the degree to which these possible relationships between the themes enhance transgender people of color's resilience to traumatic life events. [3]For instance, the majority of participants shared a critical incident in their racial/ethnic identity development where they developed a sense of racial/ethnic pride that occurred within their family network. [4]Some of these experiences were with extended family. [5]Future research might investigate these critical incidents further to understand potential resilience. [6]Additionally, participants described being in connection with other transgender people of color who also had a strong sense of racial/ethnic pride was an important source of resilience, and future research could explore this further.
Commentary
In sentence 1, the authors begin with the classification of potential relationships, and they propose two equal but different categories of those relationships—one between developing pride and family support and one between developing pride and connecting with community. There is no obvious reason that one relationship was put first and one second, which means that the authors view these as equal possibilities.

Classification is also found at the micro-level. See Table 4.5 and the commentary that accompanies for how Singh and McKleroy (2011, p. 38) used classification in their Future Research Directions and Limitations of Study section.

Of course, organizational patterns can be combined and often are. Try identifying the pattern or patterns used by analyzing the excerpt from Choi and Miller's (2014, pp. 340–341) literature review and answering the questions that accompany it in Practice Exercise 4.2. You can check your answers in the Appendix.

PRACTICE EXERCISE 4.2. Identifying Organizational Patterns

TEXT

[1]An emerging body of research suggests that stigma toward counseling occurs across three distinct domains (Ludwikowski et al., 2009; Vogel et al., 2006, 2007; Vogel, Wade, & Ascheman, 2009). [2]*Public stigma* refers to an individual's perception of societal stigma related to seeking counseling (Corrigan, 2004; Komiya, Good, & Sherrod, 2000). [3]*Stigma by close others* refers to an individual's perception of stigma toward counseling held by members of their close social network (Vogel, Wade, et al., 2009). [4]Stigma by close others

construct was originally developed because an individual's experience with stigma toward counseling among close peers, family members, or friends may differ from their experiences of stigma in the general population (Vogel, Wade, et al., 2009). [5]*Self-stigma* refers to an individual's belief that she or he is socially unacceptable because of seeking counseling; ultimately this can have a detrimental impact on self-esteem (Vogel et al., 2006).

COMMENTARY

1. Based only on sentence 1, what organizational pattern do the authors intend to follow? How do you know?
2. Based on the terms italicized in sentences 2, 3, and 5, are the authors following the pattern they established in sentence 1? Explain.
3. Compare the italicized terms in sentences 2, 3, and 5. How do these terms compare to one another? Why did the authors present them in this order? How is their decision related to organizational patterns?

The Language of Classification

Just as writers use language to support readers' recognition of hierarchical organizational patterns, they also use it to support readers' recognition of classification. For example, when introducing a classification pattern, writers will typically use more general or abstract terms, and they will propose classifications of these terms into nonspecific classifications such as *types, kinds, varieties, categories, groups, elements, parts, domains, factors, elements*, and so on. They may specify the number of specific classifications that exist (e.g., three domains), or they may simply say that there are *many, various, numerous, several, a variety of*, or *a number of* so that they can use terms that imply a selection on their part. If writers want to imply a selection, it is likely that they are moving to a hierarchical order wherein they can use such terms as *the most* or *the primary*.

Typically, classification includes a great deal of definition, as writers must define and explain their classifications. Consequently, classification arguments usually include such terms as *refer to, comprise, is composed of, include, consist of, mean, is defined as, is characterized by*, and so on. And, of course, the use of more concrete or specific vocabulary and expanded noun phrases also supports classification, as the writers break down the larger category into smaller categories.

Parallelism is one aspect of language structure that is a fundamental aspect of academic writing in general, irrespective of the organizational pattern that one chooses. However, parallelism is especially relevant to classification. Parallelism may be and, in fact, should be used at all levels of academic writing. Parallelism refers to the idea that once writers have established that they are following a particular pattern, they need to make it easy for readers to follow the pattern. From a structural point of view, this means that writers need to use vocabulary that is the appropriate "weight" (i.e., abstract, concrete, general, specific) for the pattern. This also means that they need to follow the same grammatical construction. In addition, this means that they need to maintain the order that they established at the beginning of the pattern. See excerpts from Singh and McKleroy (2011, p. 38) and Choi and Miller (2014, pp. 340–341) in Tables 4.6 and 4.7, respectively, and the commentary that accompanies them for an explanation of how parallelism is used to support the organizational pattern at different levels.

Cause–Effect

Within the overarching, problem–conclusion structure of academic research writing, you will find that cause–effect organizational patterns are also quite common. Identifying a problem and arguing a conclusion inherently suggests that a writer would necessarily engage in some discussion of causes and effects as part of her argumentation. Cause–effect organization can be a pattern at any level, but it is perhaps more usual to see it used in combination with hierarchical organization or classification. See Table 4.8 for a discussion of how Choi and Miller (2014, pp. 340–341) use a cause–effect pattern in combination with both classification and hierarchical organizational patterns.

TABLE 4.6. Parallelism at the Macro-Level

Text

Singh and McKleroy (2011, p. 38) use a classification organization pattern for their findings and implications. Their themes are classified in the following categories:

- Pride in one's gender and ethnic/racial identity
- Recognizing and negotiating gender and racial/ethnic oppression
- Navigating relationships with family
- Accessing health care and financial resources
- Connecting with an activist transgender community of color
- Cultivating spirituality and hope for the future

Commentary

As you can see, each category is represented by an expanded noun phrase. Except for the first category, all of the noun phrases begin with gerunds (i.e., verbs that have become nouns through the addition of -ing). In a perfect world, the first category would also begin with a gerund. However, the verb that would accompany pride is *have,* and while *have* can be a gerund, it is unusual to use it that way in academic writing language. Thus the authors have used parallel structure insofar as they can.

TABLE 4.7. Parallelism at the Micro-Level

Text

Choi and Miller (2014, pp. 340–341) combine classification and hierarchical organizational patterns in their literature review.

[1]An emerging body of research suggests that <u>stigma toward counseling</u> occurs across three distinct domains (Ludwikowski et al., 2009; Vogel et al., 2006, 2007; Vogel, Wade, & Ascheman, 2009). [2]*Public stigma* refers to an individual's perception of societal stigma related to seeking counseling (Corrigan, 2004; Komiya, Good, & Sherrod, 2000). [3]*Stigma by close others* refers to an individual's perception of stigma toward counseling held by members of their close social network (Vogel, Wade, et al., 2009). [4]Stigma by close others construct was originally developed because an individual's experience with stigma toward counseling among close peers, family members, or friends may differ from their experiences of stigma in the general population (Vogel, Wade, et al., 2009). [5]*Self-stigma* refers to an individual's belief that she or he is socially unacceptable because of seeking counseling; ultimately this can have a detrimental impact on self-esteem (Vogel et al., 2006).

Commentary

Notice how the pattern established with the first domain in sentence 2—domain name + "refers to" + noun phrase that includes referring to an individual—is repeated in sentences 3 and 5 for each new domain. The grammatical construction for defining each domain is almost identical, even though the words are slightly different. Repetition of grammatical constructions in this way is a strategy that academic writers can and should use often to increase the coherence of any organization pattern they use.

TABLE 4.8. Hierarchical, Classification, and Cause–Effect Organization Patterns

Text	Commentary
Stigma toward counseling is an especially relevant construct for AAPI populations, who tend to report higher levels of stigma toward seeking counseling than other cultural groups (Gilbert et al., 2007).	This claim appears in sentence 4 of the first paragraph of the subsection. The paragraph follows a hierarchical organizational pattern. This claim represents the most specific claim of the paragraph.
An emerging body of research suggests that <u>stigma toward counseling</u> occurs across three distinct domains (Ludwikowski et al., 2009; Vogel et al., 2006, 2007; Vogel, Wade, & Ascheman, 2009).	This sentence begins the second paragraph of the subsection. It introduces a paragraph organized by both classification and hierarchy. Classification is indicated by the reference to "three distinct domains." The manner in which the domains are later expressed indicates a hierarchical order from bigger to smaller. The domains are defined in order as public stigma, stigma by close others, and self-stigma.

(continued)

TABLE 4.8. *(continued)*

Text	Commentary
Third paragraph in full [1]Current theory and research suggest that public stigma and stigma by close others <u>influence</u> attitudes toward seeking professional help (i.e., an individual's broad feelings about seeking assistance from mental health professionals when facing emotional and relational challenges that are not dependent upon particular kinds of distress or types of professionals) <u>indirectly through</u> self-stigma toward counseling (Fischer & Farina, 1995; Kim & Omizo, 2003; Ludwikowski et al., 2009; Vogel et al., 2006). [2]Research also demonstrates the <u>indirect way</u> in which public stigma <u>relates to</u> willingness through self-stigma and attitudes (Vogel et al., 2007). [3]The <u>influence</u> of perceived public stigma and stigma by close others on an individual's self-stigma toward counseling seems especially salient for AAPI populations, <u>who tend to be</u> apprehensive about deviating from societal and close network norms (Kim et al., 1999; Yang et al., 2007). [4]<u>However</u>, this body of research is <u>based on primarily</u> European American samples (although one recent study by Cheng, Kwan, & Sevig, 2013 examined the relationship between stigma by close others and self-stigma toward counseling with a sample of racially diverse college students); <u>therefore the generalizability</u> of these findings <u>regarding the relationships</u> between stigma domains and willingness to seek counseling across AAPI populations is unclear.	Sentence 1 of the third paragraph introduces the claim that the three domains classified in paragraph 2 are related to each other and are causes that have an effect on attitudes toward counseling. According to the sentence, domain 1 and domain 2 join together to indirectly influence attitudes vis-à-vis domain 3. Notice that sentence 1 uses parallelism by mentioning the three domains from paragraph 2 in the same order that they are mentioned in that paragraph. Sentence 2 from the authors adds to the claim by citing evidence that two of the domains are also causes that have an effect on willingness. According to the sentence, domain 1 indirectly affects willingness through domain 3. Again, the authors use parallelism by maintaining the order of the domains (i.e., 1 is before 3). In sentences 1 and 2, the authors are establishing their general claim that stigma has an effect on counseling. Sentence 3 links the established cause–effect relationship to the authors' more specific claim that stigma affects the AAPI population's attitude toward counseling. In addition, sentence 3 proposes a reason for that effect by providing additional information about the AAPI population's relationship with social (i.e., domain 1) and close network (i.e., domain 2) groups. Notice again how the authors maintain parallelism in using the domains. Thus, in these four sentences, you can clearly see the interplay between problem–conclusion, hierarchical, classification, and cause–effect organization patterns. The entire subsection is structured to demonstrate that a problem exists. Hierarchical organization is used to guide readers to accept specific claims in paragraphs 1 and 2. Classification is used in paragraph 2 to break one concept from the claim into smaller concepts. Cause–effect is used in paragraph 3 to discuss the cause–effect relationships between the smaller concepts and the claim and to finally illustrate that the problem is real.

TABLE 4.9. Signal Words or Phrases for Cause–Effect Organization

Conjunctions and other expressions	Verbs	Transitions	Nouns
because because of due to for this reason as a result	cause create produce result in stem from affect lead to influence	consequently therefore thus accordingly	reason effect results consequence

Language Use

As indicated, cause–effect organization uses parallelism to help the reader follow the logic of the writer's argument. Without parallelism, readers have trouble processing cause–effect relationships, particularly when there are multiple or interacting causes or effects, as is often the case in research writing. Cause–effect organization is also supported by signal words or phrases, including the brief list provided in Table 4.9, as well as many others.

Especially with transition words, be cautious that you do not overuse them. If you know you tend to overuse a certain transition word (e.g., *moreover*), then be on the lookout for those words when you are proofreading. Now that you have an idea of the most common thought and expression patterns in academic research writing, spend some time noticing how often those patterns are used and how those patterns are expressed in your discipline and your own writing. You can get started by completing Practice Exercises 4.3 and 4.4.

PRACTICE EXERCISE 4.3. Noticing Thought and Expression Patterns in Your Discipline

1. Select any three research articles in your discipline.
2. Analyze the macro-level structure (i.e., titles and organization of sections and subsections).
   a. Do you see evidence of hierarchical, classification, or cause–effect organizational patterns?
   b. Do you see evidence of parallelism?
3. Look at the literature review or a subsection of the literature review. If it

is a subsection, you are looking for one with more than one paragraph. Analyze the meso-level structure (i.e., order of the paragraphs).

   a. Do you see evidence of hierarchical, classification, or cause–effect organizational patterns in the order of the paragraphs?

4. Look through all three articles. Find instances of hierarchical, classification, and cause–effect organizational patterns at the micro-level (i.e., order of sentences in a paragraph) in those articles. You should be able to find all three in most articles.

   a. Underline the words in the sentences that help you to know the organizational pattern. Think about the vocabulary continua, noun phrases, signal words and phrases, and parallelism.

PRACTICE EXERCISE 4.4. Analyzing the Structure of Your Text

- Select a piece of writing you have done that is complete.

- On day 1, list your basic argument and your macro-level structure headings and subheadings in a blank document. When you had the opportunity to "freely" organize sections and subsections, what organizational pattern did you follow? (Remember that some sections and subsections are simply required, so you may not have been able to "freely" organize very much.) Do you remember why you followed that pattern? If you had the opportunity to change your macro-level structure, would you? Why or why not?

- On day 2, begin analyzing your writing section by section for meso-level structure. For each section that contains more than one paragraph, ask yourself what the relationship is between the paragraphs. Can you classify the order of your paragraphs according to one of the organizational patterns we discussed? What language (i.e., vocabulary or grammar) do you use at the beginning or end of each paragraph that helps readers to know how the paragraphs are related? Do you think readers would find it easy or hard to explain the relationship between your paragraphs? Explain. If they would find it hard, what do you need to change?

- On day 3, or whenever you finish your meso-level analysis, select specific paragraphs from your writing for an analysis of micro-level structure. For each paragraph you select, number the sentences in the paragraph. Read the whole paragraph and ask yourself what the paragraph is trying to achieve (i.e., what is the purpose of the paragraph?). Does the paragraph achieve this purpose? If yes, how does the structural organization of the paragraph contribute to the paragraph's achieving its purpose? If no or maybe not, ask yourself how each sentence relates to the previous sentence from a structural perspective. Are there structural gaps—relationships between sentences that are not clear? If yes, what is missing? Remember, look at it like a reader, not like a writer. What is clear to you as the writer may not be clear to someone else as the reader.

CHAPTER SUMMARY AND REMINDERS

As we have said in this chapter, we want you to gain a deeper understanding of how the structure of academic language reflects the preferred thought patterns of academic readers. We hope that you understand the organizational patterns involved in translating thought to words a bit better now and that you have some ideas for how to improve your use of coherent structure. We are including a reminder list of awareness and action suggestions from this chapter in Summary Table 4.1 so that you have a handy place to refer to them quickly.

SUMMARY TABLE 4.1. AWARENESS AND ACTION REMINDERS

Be aware . . .	Take action . . .
Writers and readers are roles, not people—the writer is the persuader and the reader is the doubter.	See writing as having three levels: the macro-, meso-, and micro-levels.
Academic writers have a heightened sense of audience awareness.	Become familiar with the organizational patterns that are most common in academic writing.
Academic writing is writer-responsible.	Learn how to predict the reader's thought process.
A coherent structure is logical, clear, and orderly.	Expand your vocabulary to support your use of different organizational patterns.
Writers must write for the readers' expectations and sense of coherence, not their own.	Use parallel structure *always*!

CHAPTER 5

The Use of Tone and Style in Your Academic Writing

In Chapter 4, we discussed writer–reader roles in academic writing and how they have contributed to the heightened sense of audience awareness that is characteristic of academic writing. We also discussed how this audience awareness results from the writer-responsible expectations that are fundamental to academic writing. We elaborated on how writer–reader roles, audience awareness, and writer-responsible expectations are related to both the structure of thoughts and the language of expression in academic writing. In particular, we focused on what counts as coherent structure in academic writing and how writers create and use coherent structure.

Our awareness and action foci remain the same for this chapter. For our **awareness focus**, we still want you to gain a deeper understanding of how academic writing language is specifically related to writer–reader roles. For our **action focus**, we still provide ideas for steps that you can take to increase your familiarity with the thought patterns underlying the language and develop your ability to use them. However, in this chapter, we focus on rational tone and cohesive style, which are two additional essential characteristics of academic writing. Each of these characteristics is related to the writer's imagined interactions with the reader and her attempts to anticipate, mitigate, or circumvent readers' objections so that readers will be persuaded to consider the writer's argument as sound, logical, and credible.

RATIONAL TONE

In writing, tone is the writer's attitude toward the reader and the topic about which he is writing. The writer's tone influences readers to perceive the writer and the topic in a certain way. For example, a writer's sarcastic tone may influence some readers to perceive him as funny, but it may influence other readers to perceive him as negative, pessimistic, or mean.

In academic writing, a rational tone is preferred. Rational means that the writer is expected to present herself through writing as having a neutral, impersonal, and reasonable attitude toward the reader. Writers are expected to present an attitude that demonstrates that they believe the reader to be a qualified and fair-minded evaluator of their ideas. The writer is not necessarily expected to have a neutral attitude toward the topic, because, of course, she is trying to make some kind of argument about it. However, the writer is expected to have a mostly impersonal and logical attitude toward the topic. For example, the writer's attitude toward the topic should include an acknowledgement that there are other valid perspectives on the topic that may contradict her own.

Given that writers are persuaders and readers are doubters, the obvious point of using a rational tone in academic writing is to allow writers to create a relationship with readers that will perhaps influence readers to give writers the benefit of the doubt in cases in which readers may be inclined to find flaws. Also, using a rational tone may assist writers by helping them to convince readers that their arguments are logical (i.e., if the tone is logical, the argument must be logical). We discuss three common strategies that writers use to achieve a rational tone: hedging, signal phrases, and metacommentary.

Hedging

Hedging is the act of expressing your attitude or ideas in tentative or cautious ways. Hedging includes the use of verbs, adjectives, adverbs, nouns, and other grammatical constructions that soften the stance of the writer or decrease the strength of his claims by introducing hesitation, uncertainty, or doubt to any degree. Hedging is very common in academic writing. In fact, we came across an unsubstantiated claim as we were writing this section that 1 in every 100 words in good academic writing is a hedge. Although we do not know if this has ever been empirically proven, the excerpt from Choi and Miller (2014, p. 348) in Box 5.1 contains 122 words and includes six examples of hedging (see the underlined words and phrases).

Hedging is common in academic writing for a number of reasons. One of those reasons is related to the purposes and ethics of scientific research. Scientists of all types are in the business of seeking "objective truth" (i.e., empirically proven facts). However, scholars of all types—those who believe in objective truths and those who do not—understand that one of the ethical principles of science is that any claim must be proven. They also understand that one study alone does not prove a claim. Therefore, hedging is the ethical recognition that one's own findings are but one step in *possibly* proving a claim. Hedging is also the ethical recognition that

---

BOX 5.1. Example of Hedging in Claims

These findings <u>suggest</u> that Asian Americans who adhere to European cultural values place a particular emphasis on self-enhancement and growth. As a result, they <u>may view</u> counseling as an appropriate tool for self-exploration, and this perception <u>can lead</u> to lower levels of public stigma toward seeking counseling. One <u>tentative</u> explanation for this finding, in the context of AAPI individuals' bicultural context, <u>might be</u> that aspects of European American cultural values such as individualism and self-reliance are manifestations of AAPI individuals' concurrent desire to not burden one's cultural group (Triandis, McCusker, & Hui, 1990). In other words, AAPI individuals who espouse European American cultural values <u>might be</u> more willing to seek counseling so that they will not be burdensome to their family members.

---

scientific "truths" of any given moment do not necessarily remain constant. The accepted "truths" of one moment in time will not necessarily be the "truths" of another.

In addition, hedging is a useful way for writers not only to offset the readers' doubting role but also to address the fact that writers may be writing for readers who know more about the topic than they do. By using hedges, writers can demonstrate to readers that they, too, recognize that there are uncertainties and unknowns in their argument that may affect its overall strength. This reasonableness on the part of writers may influence readers to be more accepting of their arguments, because readers do not feel as though writers are ignoring obvious weaknesses. Hedging is important because, as scholars, we know that much of science seeks a truth that is "objective"; however, there are also limitations in "proving" this objective truth. Therefore, hedging recognizes this conundrum: We seek a version of the truth as scholars in our research activities; yet, when we discuss our research, we must acknowledge the limitations of our endeavors. In addition, we have to acknowledge that the theories and research activities we are currently using may not hold up forever. The history of the research in every discipline provides a clear indication that what is believed to be "true" at any given point in time is subject to change, so whatever writers may think they have uncovered or found is also subject to change over time. People once had theories about the world being flat, and we know now that is simply not true. So hedging allows us to recognize the current and future limitations of our research. We say a study's findings "suggest" something rather than "demonstrate" or "prove" something.

In Table 5.1, you can see that we have included a brief list of hedging words. This list is by no means exhaustive, and we encourage you to build your hedging vocabulary by Googling "hedging words" or "hedging and

TABLE 5.1. Hedging Words and Expressions	
Hedges are any words or expressions that show hesitation, uncertainty, or doubt to any degree on the part of the writer with respect to their claims. Examples of hedging include the following:	
Modal verbs	*may, might, can, could, would, should*
Other verbs	*appear, include, seem, believe, suppose, presume, tend*
Nouns	*possibility, probability, likelihood, tendency, assumption, claim, suggestion*
Adjectives	*possible, likely, unlikely, many, few, some, several, most, potential, considerable*
Adverbs	*probably, possibly, likely, presumably, perhaps, somewhat, largely, mostly, potentially, evidently, convincingly, debatably, apparently, hypothetically, often, occasionally, usually, generally*
Expressions	*in general; if true, then . . . ; unless*

academic writing." Most of all, we encourage you to use hedging often in your writing and to begin to notice and identify when writers in your field use hedging and when they don't. Give this kind of noticing a try in Practice Exercise 5.1 with the excerpt from Kuhlen, Galati, and Brennan (2012, pp. 37–38). You can check your answers in the Appendix.

PRACTICE EXERCISE 5.1. When to Hedge and Why

TEXT

[1]Our findings are <u>consistent with</u> the previous analysis of the speech that accompanied these gestures (Kuhlen and Brennan 2010). [2]In that study, speakers spent more time in the interaction when speakers' expectations matched addressees' feedback. [3]This <u>parallels</u> our current finding that speakers also produce more gestures per narrative element in these conditions, <u>strengthening our interpretation</u> that speakers put more effort into narrating when their expectations of their addressees are matched by addressees' behavior in the interaction. [3]Kuhlen and Brennan also found that when (and only when) speakers narrated to attentive addressees whom they had also expected to be attentive, they used more additional narrative details; in the current study, they used more peripheral gestures as well. [4]Together, these adjustments <u>suggest</u> that speakers did not produce gestures in the periphery of their gesture space to attract their addressees' attention. [5]Instead, these gestures <u>may simply</u> go hand in hand with a more vivid or engaged style of narrating. [6]Having an attentive addressee is not enough by itself to lead to a vivid narration: expecting an attentive addressee is also necessary. [7]Both of these <u>apparently</u> lead to a more engaged, and therefore a more coordinated, interaction.

QUESTIONS

1. What is the purpose of the expression "consistent with" in sentence 1? Why is it considered a hedging phrase?
2. Considering the overall meaning of sentence 2, why doesn't it contain hedging?
3. What is the purpose of the verb "parallels" in sentence 3? Why is it considered a hedging word? What is the purpose of the expression "strengthening our interpretation" in sentence 3? Why is it considered a hedging phrase?
4. What is the purpose of the verb "suggest" in sentence 4? Why is it considered a hedging word?
5. What is the purpose of the expression "may simply" in sentence 5? Why is it considered a hedging expression?
6. Considering the overall meaning of sentence 6, why doesn't it contain hedging?
7. What is the purpose of the adverb "apparently" in sentence 7? Why is it considered a hedging word?

Signal Phrases

As we discussed in Chapter 3, academic writers must both fit in and stand out. They must have something unique to contribute, but they must contextualize their contributions within past research. In academic writing, past research sets the stage for any writer's argument, and all academic writing must bear multiple and visible connections to past research. For example, academic research writing generally contains multiple in-text citations, occasional footnotes, and long lists of references. The need for writers to situate themselves in past literature results in their needing to shift from one voice to another in their writing quite regularly. This kind of shifting can be confusing for readers who are primarily concerned with trying to follow one voice—that of the writer. In writer-responsible writing, which is the case of academic writing, reader confusion must be avoided. Thus academic writers must use a variety of attribution strategies to ensure that readers can easily and clearly follow shifts in voice.

Attribution is the act of letting the reader know whose voice is metaphorically speaking. Attribution may be indicated by in-text citations, quotation marks, and signal phrases. In general, in-text citations are the most common and preferred method of attribution. When writers use in-text citations or quotation marks, they are indicating that a voice other than their own is metaphorically speaking. Signal phrases are linguistic markers in sentences that may also be used to indicate that a voice other than the writer's own is speaking. Box 5.2 illustrates the three basic patterns academic writers use for signal phrases. These patterns may vary according to

> **BOX 5.2. Basic Patterns for Signal Phrases**
>
> 1. As + Surname(s) + (Year) + signal verb + comma + direct quotation or summary or paraphrase.
>
>   As Singh and McKleroy (2011) noted, the resilience experiences of transgender people of color are understudied.
>
> 2. Surname(s) + (Year) + signal verb + direct quotation or summary or paraphrase.
>
>   Singh and McKleroy (2011) proposed that there should be more studies on the resilience experiences of transgender people of color.
>
> 3. According to + Surname(s) + (Year) + comma + direct quotation or summary or paraphrase.
>
>   According to Singh and McKleroy (2011), the resilience experiences of transgender people of color are an important area for future study.

the style guidelines preferred by your discipline. In addition, the patterns shown in Box 5.2 illustrate how to use signal phrases at the beginning of sentences. However, signal phrases may be used in the middle or at the end of sentences as well.

Because academic writing relies so much on sources and because there are only three basic patterns for signal phrases, writers are challenged to avoid repeating the same signal phrase too often. To avoid this, writers intersperse the use of just in-text citations with the use of signal phrases containing in-text citations. Some writers may only use in-text citations. This is a stylistic choice that may be personal or may reflect discipline norms. Writers also try to vary the signal verbs that they use in signal phrases. By varying the verbs, they can avoid sounding like a broken record, but they can also increase the information content of their quotations, summaries, and paraphrases. You may recall that we referred to academic research writing, especially research articles, as having dense prose. By this, we meant that every sentence carries a lot of information. Signal verbs are one way in which writers increase the density of their sentences. They are also one way that writers can increase the clarity and accuracy of their reports of others' ideas. Let's take a look at a few examples:

1. Singh and McKleroy (2011) <u>wrote</u> that the resilience experiences of transgender people of color should be studied more.
2. Singh and McKleroy (2011) <u>observed</u> that the resilience experiences of transgender people of color should be studied more.

3. Singh and McKleroy (2011) <u>suggested</u> that the resilience experiences of transgender people of color should be studied more.

4. Singh and McKleroy (2011) <u>proposed</u> that the resilience experiences of transgender people of color should be studied more.

Can you see how the change in the signal verb changes the overall meaning of each sentence? Example 1 is accurate in the sense that the authors did write that the resilience experiences of transgender people of color should be studied more, but the sentence lacks any information on the authors' attitude toward the topic. Like example 1, example 2 is also accurate in the sense that this particular view on resilience and transgender people of color is an observation in their text, but the signal verb *observed* implies that this view was possibly one of many others that they expressed. This would, in fact, be an inaccurate representation of the Singh and McKleroy text. Examples 3 and 4 are also both accurate in the sense that the authors are putting forth a particular point of view, but example 3 implies that the way they put forth this idea was in the form of a suggestion, which is not accurate. Example 4 uses the word "proposed," which is accurate in both meaning and the strength of their actual claim.

In Table 5.2, you can see that we have included a brief list of signal verbs. This list is by no means exhaustive, and we encourage you to build your signal verb vocabulary by Googling "signal phrases" or "signal verbs." Most of all, we encourage you to begin noticing how writers in your discipline accomplish shifts in voice so that you will understand the various strategies you might use in your own writing. Try your hand at identifying voice shifts in the excerpt from Bugg (2013, p. 1149) in Practice Exercise 5.2. Then try determining where and why attribution of some type is necessary in the *modified* excerpt from Choi and Miller (2014, p. 341) in Practice 5.3. (Their original text has been modified to remove attribution markers.) You can check your answers in the Appendix. You will likely

TABLE 5.2. Signal Verbs

Signal verbs are verbs that you can use when referring to other voices in your writing. Signal verbs can help you to accurately convey the attitude that other voices had toward their topics. Examples of signal verbs include the following:

Neutral/weak	Medium	Strong
explain	emphasize	argue
compare	claim	assert
observe	confirm	affirm
present	suggest	propose
report	discuss	charge
describe	point to	refute
state	acknowledge	criticize

notice that identifying voice shifts and ideas that require attribution is not as easy as it seems, which will give you an idea of why it is so important that you as a writer use clear voice-shifting strategies for your readers.

PRACTICE EXERCISE 5.2. Identifying Voice Shifts

TEXT

[1]Recent work by geographers has highlighted not just the importance of theorising belonging, but also the necessity of "unpacking the ways that belonging is actively practiced" (Mee and Wright 2009:774). [2]Although diaspora studies have attended to the importance of place, scholars have challenged the ways in which current theorisations of diaspora both "ignore the reading of the landscape from the vantage point of the displaced" and "privilege mobility" while disparaging struggles for emplacement (Casteel 2007:2). [3]Thus, this work builds on growing theory on landscape and belonging, such as that by Mitchell (1997), Tolia-Kelly (2006) and Trudeau (2006), particularly in the way that national identity and belonging is contested and worked out at the local level. [4]Through the consideration of subaltern voices, the research also extends an emerging literature that opens up what Casteel (2007) has called a "critical mode of pastoral." [5]This mode emphasises the pastoral's capacity to be "simultaneously conservative and oppositional" and allows transnationals to "assert the need for place while simultaneously registering the historic realities of displacement" (Casteel 2007:13).

QUESTIONS

1. How many voice shifts do you see in sentence 1? Remember that voice shifts can be indicated by signal phrases as well as in-text citations.
2. How many voice shifts do you see in sentence 2?
3. How many voice shifts do you see in sentence 3?
4. How many voice shifts do you see in sentence 4?
5. How many voice shifts do you see in sentence 5?

PRACTICE EXERCISE 5.3. Identifying and Explaining Use of Attribution

TEXT

[1]We also extended research in this area by accounting for AAPI individuals' espousal of European American cultural values. [2]It is generally accepted that AAPI individuals in the United States exist in a bicultural context in which they

are exposed to European American culture and their culture of origin. [3]Due to this sustained exposure to both cultures, AAPI individuals may internalize aspects of Asian culture and European American culture. [4]Therefore, attending to espousal of both Asian cultural values and European American cultural values might provide a better approximation of AAPI's willingness to seek counseling. [5]For example, AAPI individuals who espouse European American values (e.g., openness and change) might feel less shame about counseling and might therefore be more willing to seeking it. [6]We hypothesized that European American cultural values would be associated with less perceived public stigma and stigma by close others. [7]In addition, although no prior studies have examined the relationship between European American cultural values and willingness to seek counseling, European American cultural values have been linked to more positive attitudes toward seeking professional help. [8]Therefore, given the established link between attitudes toward seeking professional help and willingness to seek counseling, we hypothesized that European American cultural values would relate positively to willingness to seek counseling.

QUESTIONS

1. Read through the entire excerpt. Which sentences are likely wholly or partially the authors' voice? Remember that sentences can blend voices with part of the sentence expressing the author's voice and part of the sentence expressing the voices of other researchers.
2. If you found sentences that partially include the authors' voices, which part of the sentence would need some type of attribution and why?
3. Which sentences are likely wholly the voices of other researchers? Why do you think this?
4. Are there any sentences that could go either way (i.e., they could be the authors' voices or other researchers' voices)? Why is it difficult to decide the voice of these sentences?

Metacommentary

In writer-responsible writing, writers are trying to anticipate and to some extent control readers' reactions to their texts. They are imagining the doubting reader who is questioning and challenging their argument at every turn, and they are trying to counter the questions and challenges they imagine with a logical and clear argument that contains all of the information that the reader needs to accept the argument as valid, sound, and credible. One of the strategies that writers often use to manage their doubting readers is metacommentary. Metacommentary essentially consists of instances of writers commenting *in* their text *on* their own ideas in an effort to *help* readers understand their arguments in ways that they wish.

Graff and Birkenstein (2014) compare metacommentary to a voice-over narrator in a television program or film. Their comparison highlights

TABLE 5.3. Expressions That Introduce Metacommentary				
Metacommentary expressions are expressions you can use when you want to emphasize something that you want your reader to notice, explain or clarify something about your argument for your reader, or otherwise direct your reader to understand or interpret your argument in a specific way. Examples of metacommentary expressions include the following:				
of course	*i.e. (that is)*	*essentially*	*to clarify*	*X aligns with Y*
indeed	*that is*	*ultimately*	*to explain*	*X echoes Y*
arguably	*in other words*	*what I/we mean*	*which means*	*X contradicts Y*
undeniably	*to put it another way*	*by this I/we mean*	*meaning . . .*	*X challenges Y*

the fact that the writer role can be subdivided between the roles of writer and narrator. The writer is intent on communicating a clear and logical argument, while the narrator is intent on being sure that the audience understands what the writer is doing. Metacommentary is the voice of the narrator entering into the writer's argument to direct the audience's understanding of what the writer is doing.

Writers can use metacommentary to emphasize things that they think are important for the reader to notice at a specific moment in the text, to share their thought process of how ideas fit together with readers, to explain or clarify the meaning of their statements and ideas, and to share their intentions with readers. The hope of writers when using metacommentary is that the additional insight they provide for readers through the metacommentary will induce readers to develop expectations and interpretations that are in alignment with those that writers want them to have. In Table 5.3, we have included a brief list of a few expressions that may be used to introduce metacommentary. We encourage you to begin looking for metacommentary in the excerpts from Walker-Williams, van Eeden, and van der Merwe (2012, p. 619) and Singh and McKleroy (2011, p. 40) of Practice Exercise 5.4. See the Appendix for our answers.

PRACTICE EXERCISE 5.4. Noticing Metacommentary in Academic Writing

Read each text. Underline or list the words/expressions that you think are examples of metacommentary. Then decide why the author may have decided to use this metacommentary: to emphasize, to explain or clarify, or to direct readers' understanding. You may check your answers in the Appendix.

TEXT 1

The pattern of disclosure of participants in this study corresponds to what is reported in literature, namely that family members, mothers and professionals are the most likely sources of support when disclosing (Sauzier, 1989).

About half of the participants were treated for a mood disorder, which is supported by literature reporting that the long-term effects of CSA frequently include a range of symptoms such as depression (Allen, 2008; Bennett & Hughes, 2000; Finkelhor & Browne, 1986; Spies, 2006a). The most frequently reported effects of CSA are of an emotional nature. Victims of CSA experience emotions of degradation and humiliation leading to low self-esteem (Saffy, 2003). This also seems evident in the findings that just below half of the participants experienced trust as the most prominent difficulty after the abuse, about a third experienced poor intimacy and relationships, and a quarter experienced poor self-esteem. Distortions in attachment that result from sexual abuse in childhood can be toxic in all future relationships, and especially so in the areas of self-esteem, intimacy, trust and the ability to bond (Taylor & Thomas, 2003). All four traumagenic dynamics were experienced by more than half of the women and the rest experienced at least a combination of two of the dynamics. This illustrates indeed the severe and unique psychological impact of the CSA experience as reported by the authors Finkelhor and Browne (1986).

TEXT 2

Finally, the finding that participants accessed their spirituality as a source of resilience—which then led to increased hope about their future as transgender people of color—is similar to other qualitative investigations of racial/ethnic minorities who have survived traumatic life events (Singh, 2006; Stevens, 1997). Investigations of trauma and spirituality are not necessarily new to the trauma field. However, recent literature has emphasized that practitioners should explore survivors' spiritual beliefs, especially if spirituality is a social location that assists survivors in making meaning of trauma and resilience they have experienced (Brown, 2008; Hartling, 2004). Participants particularly shared that their sense of spiritual resilience was more salient than their religious coping. This finding echoes Kidd and Witten's (2009) study of aging transgender persons' spiritual beliefs. In this study, the authors found participants' belief systems were often nontraditional and encouraged practitioners to "be aware of the diverse and non-traditional nature of belief structures and how these mediate life course development and impact late and end of life struggles" (p. 62). Overall, findings of the current study call for practitioners to address how contextual factors and multiple identities intersect and influence the well-being of transgender people of color's experiences of traumatic life events (Mizock & Lewis, 2008; Nemoto et al., 2004).

COHESIVE STYLE

In writing, style is the way that something is written. It is one of the ways that writers express their personalities and voices. For example, a writer may have a flowery style, which means that she "decorates" her writing with complex or complicated words or grammar to try to make it look more sophisticated for the reader. Readers may be impressed or put off by a flowery style, depending on their own personalities and the expectations they have of the type of text they are reading. Undergraduate students sometimes try to impress professors with flowery style, hoping that the style will compensate for minimal ideas or a lack of coherence.

In academic writing, a cohesive style is preferred. Cohesive means that ideas are linguistically linked to one another so that readers can follow the writer's thought progression. Although some elements of cohesive style can be found at the macro-level, cohesive style is primarily a characteristic that affects the meso- and micro-levels of writing.

At the macro-level, texts are often divided into sections and subsections that have headings. These headings more or less eliminate the need for writers to connect ideas linguistically between sections; the heading does the work of shifting from one topic to another for the writer. However, writers can use cohesive devices to either connect to a previous section or project to a subsequent section. For example, the following sentence was the first sentence of the Research Methods section of Hawkins, Manzi, and Ojeda (2014, p. 331): "To learn more about these embodied and gendered processes of how we become geographers and academics throughout our time in graduate school and beyond, we decided to use our own lives and the lives of our colleagues, friends and families as inspiration." The use of *these* as a definite article functions as a directional cue to the reader, directing the reader to understand that the "embodied and gendered processes" discussed in this sentence were already introduced in the previous section.

Although cohesive devices may or may not be used between sections with headings, there is frequently some type of cohesion between the conclusion and the introduction of academic texts. Because writers are leading readers to see their research gap or problem in the way that they themselves see it, they inevitably return to the gap or problem in the conclusion. Thus writers may use cohesive devices in their conclusions to remind readers of the link between their gap and their conclusion. For example, the excerpts from Singh and McKleroy (2011, pp. 34, 42) in Box 5.3 include cohesive devices that link the conclusion to the research gap from the introduction. See Box 5.3 and the commentary that follows it for further explanation.

The words and ideas that are linked between the research gap of the introduction and the conclusion have been detailed in Table 5.4. The types of cohesion devices used by the authors to create the links have also been included in the table.

At the meso-level, cohesion is used to link paragraphs, and this type of linking is fairly common in both backward and forward directions in academic writing. In fact, you can see how Walker-Williams and colleagues (2012, p. 617) did this in one of the subsections of their literature review in Box 5.4. Notice how the last sentence of the first paragraph introduces the topic of posttraumatic growth and the first sentence of the second paragraph begins with a definition of that term.

> **BOX 5.3. Macro-Level Cohesion between the Conclusion and the Introduction**
>
> **Introduction**
>
> The purpose of this study was to explore the resilience processes used by transgender people of color to cope with traumatic events and to provide explicit clinical implications relevant for mental health providers working with this group.
>
> **Conclusion**
>
> This phenomenological and feminist study explored the resilience processes transgender people of color have despite the additive stressors of racism and transphobia related to experiencing traumatic life events. In general, transgender people of color negotiate multiple identities that have been historically marginalized. Therefore, ethical and affirmative practice with survivors of traumatic life events must also address issues of health care, employment, and interpersonal support systems. Practitioners may also recognize the important role they may take in not only validating the experiences of trauma and resilience for transgender people of color, but also in playing an integral role in increasing societal awareness, acceptance, and respect for transgender people of color.

At the micro-level, cohesion is actually used in two ways. On the one hand, it links sentences to one another. On the other hand, it links ideas within a sentence with each other. We present and discuss several examples of both of these links later in this chapter.

In writer-responsible writing, a cohesive style is very important, because writers are not supposed to expect readers to "read between the lines" or "figure it out." Rather, writers are supposed to spell out the exact links between ideas so that readers understand the connection between the writers' thoughts. Often, when discussing cohesion, writers talk about the "flow" of their writing. By this, they mean their ability to create smooth and logical links between ideas so that their argument vis-à-vis their writing flows smoothly like water flowing down a river.

Creating flow is not easy because it requires the writer to see the argument through the eyes of the reader, which means that the writer has to anticipate what is known and unknown to the reader in terms of the content of ideas. It also means that the writer has to know what assumptions are allowable according to the reader. Allowable assumptions are connections that the reader can and will make that do not require intentional linking on the part of the writer. New writers are often surprised at how few

TABLE 5.4. Analysis of Macro-Level Cohesion between the Introduction and Conclusion

Research gap of the Introduction	Conclusion	Cohesion devices
"explore the resilience processes"	• "explored the resilience processes" • "resilience"	• Exact repetition • Substitution by variation on original word or phrase
"transgender people of color"	• "transgender people of color" (four repetitions)	• Exact repetition
"traumatic events"	• "traumatic life events" (two repetitions) • "trauma"	• Exact repetition • Substitution by variation on original word or phrase
"transgender people of color to cope with traumatic events"	• "survivors of traumatic life events"	• Substitution by categorical noun
"explicit clinical implications"	• "ethical and affirmative practice" • "issues of health care, employment, and interpersonal support systems" • "important role they may take in not only validating the experiences" • "playing an integral role in increasing societal awareness, acceptance, and respect"	• Substitution by elaboration (all)
"mental health providers"	• Practitioners	• Substitution by categorical noun

BOX 5.4. Meso-Level Cohesion

Last sentence of paragraph 1

Aldwin (1994) refers to this as transformational coping, which the authors Tedeschi and Calhoun (2004a, p. 1) have expanded on and termed "posttraumatic growth."

First sentence of paragraph 2

Posttraumatic growth is defined as the "positive psychological change experienced as a result of the struggle with highly challenging life crises" (Tedeschi & Calhoun, 2004a, p. 1).

assumptions are allowable and how much cohesion is required in academic writing.

Because cohesion is so important to the writer–reader relationship in academic writing, there are many ways that it can be created using cohesive devices. We discuss three categories—repetition, reader cues, and grammar—that each include multiple cohesion devices.

Repetition

By far, the most common way of achieving cohesion in academic writing is through some form of repetition. As we have discussed, readers are not expected to work that hard when reading an academic text; everything is supposed to flow and be easy to follow. This means that readers are also not expected to remember and hold information for very long as they read, because this makes reading harder. Consequently, writers must repeat the topics and the points they are trying to make very frequently. Readers should not be required to remember a writer's topic for more than one to two sentences without some kind of reminder.

Because readers are not required to remember information for very long, academic writing at the micro-level of sentences within a paragraph follows a pattern of introducing a topic or idea in one sentence, then repeating that topic or idea in some way in the next sentence while introducing some new information. In the sentence after that, the new information is repeated, and some other new information is added. This repeat-old-information-add-new-information pattern continues to the end of the paragraph. In addition, there are always some topics or ideas that are considered key words or ideas that may be repeated in some way throughout the entire paragraph because the writer wants to be sure that the reader is following his argument. We will see how this repeat-old-information-add-new-information technique is used in various examples as we discuss different cohesive devices that assist writers in creating this pattern.

Repetition in academic writing can be achieved in two ways—exact repetition and repetition through substitution.

Exact Repetition

As we just mentioned, there are always some key words or terms that are repeated verbatim throughout an entire text or a paragraph. These key words or terms are usually introduced at the beginning of the text or paragraph, and they are key because they are the words or terms that the reader needs to really notice and understand in order to follow your argument. Let's begin by considering a whole research article. The article by Kuhlen and colleagues (2012) is 20 pages long without the abstract, appendices, and references. The text of those pages contains 8,435 words. The focus is on gestures, and gesturing is part of the title of the article. The word *gesture* appears 244 times, *gestures* appears 92 times, *gesturing* appears 22 times, and *gestured* appears 18 times for a total of 376 occurrences. This means that, mathematically, some variation on the word *gesture* appears 18.8 times on every page. That's a lot, and that's normal in academic writing! Although you may feel like you are repeating yourself excessively and unnecessarily as you write, you actually must repeat certain words over and over to have a cohesive style in academic writing.

Let's see how this works at the paragraph level now. The excerpt from Gould, Dariotis, Mendelson, and Greenberg (2012, p. 969) in Box 5.5 contains 146 words and four sentences. In that span of words, the following words from the first sentence are repeated multiple times: *yoga* (four times), *mindfulness* (three times), *techniques* (two times), *contemplative* (two times), and *self-regulation* (two times).

Substitution

In addition to exact repetition, cohesion may also be created through the use of words that closely approximate key words. These words replace the key word or idea, but they do so in a way that reminds the reader of the key word. They are not so different that the reader thinks the writer is introducing a new idea. There are several different kinds of substitution: variations on a word, synonyms, pronouns, categorical nouns, ellipsis, and elaboration.

BOX 5.5. Repetition of Key Words in a Paragraph

Mindfulness practices that utilize yoga and other contemplative techniques are a promising approach for enhancing key aspects of self-regulation (e.g., Chiesa & Serretti, 2009; Greenberg & Harris, 2011; Lutz et al., 2009; Tang et al., 2009). Derived from Eastern contemplative traditions, *mindfulness* involves attending to the present moment in a sustained and receptive fashion (Brown & Ryan, 2003). Yoga, a specific form of mindfulness, involves maintaining focused attention on one's breath and body while performing movements that improve strength and flexibility. Indeed, the Sanskrit root of "yoga" means "to yoke, to join, and to direct and concentrate one's attention" (Collins, 1998, p. 564). Yoga and other meditative techniques have been shown to increase attention and self-regulation and reduce stress and improve functioning in adults (Arias, Steinberg, Banga, & Trestment, 2006; Kirkwood et al., 2005; Ospina et al., 2007; Pilkington, Kirkwood, Rampes, & Richardson, 2005; Shapiro, Brown, & Biegel, 2007).

VARIATIONS ON A WORD

Words have many forms. One of the easiest things that writers can do to ensure that they are repeating key words without sounding monotonous is to use variations on the same word. For example, if a word has a noun form, a verb form, and an adjective form, the writer can use all of these. The previously discussed example from Kuhlen et al. (2012) regarding the use of variations on *gesture* illustrates how variations on a word may be used to create cohesion. Obviously, using the dictionary to find out the options available to you as a writer is useful for understanding the possible variations.

SYNONYMS

Synonyms are words that more or less have the same meaning. People often think that synonyms have the same meaning as the words they replace, but all words have some differences in how they are used in different contexts. This is where using synonyms can become tricky. Using a synonym to achieve repetition may work provided that you choose words the reader understands as synonyms. However, if you choose words that the reader does not recognize as synonyms, you will create confusion. Thus it is best to use exact repetition or variations on a word if you are not certain about the synonym. The dictionary, the thesaurus, and even the word processing program you use can provide you with ideas for synonyms. We would like to offer a word of caution about trying to use synonyms for terms that are agreed-upon terms in your field. Often, there is no acceptable synonym for a specific agreed-upon term in a specific field. Any attempt to use a synonym would result in confusion, because other members of your discipline-specific CoP would *not* recognize that you are using a synonym. They might mistakenly think that you are introducing a new idea, which would inevitably lead to confusion.

PRONOUNS

Pronouns are words such as *it, him, her, them, this,* and *these* that take the place of nouns. In speaking, we use pronouns a lot, and this works fine because we are often either speaking with people who share our immediate context, so that gestures and other nonverbal signals can be used for clarification, or with someone with whom we have familiarity, so that we can follow what she is saying through our previous knowledge of that person. In academic writing, it may be tempting to use pronouns, but in general, it should be avoided—not eliminated but avoided. As we mentioned earlier, readers are supposed to find following the writer's argument easy, and they are not supposed to have to remember and hold information for very long. Every time a writer uses a pronoun, the reader has to remember the noun to which the pronoun refers. In addition, pronouns can become confusing if the pronoun refers to a plural subject but there is another plural noun between the subject and the pronoun. In general, we would say that it is okay to introduce a noun and use a pronoun in the very next sentence, but in the third sentence, you should return to the noun by repeating it in some way other than a pronoun. Notice how the excerpt from Bugg (2013, p. 1149) in Box 5.6 follows this pattern. The words to notice have been underlined.

CATEGORICAL NOUNS

We are using the term *categorical nouns* to refer to cases in which a broad or general category such as *problem* or *situation* is used to substitute for a previously mentioned idea. Categorical nouns are more general or more abstract than the word or idea that they are replacing. Often these categorical nouns are accompanied by a directional cue such as *this* or *these* that reminds the reader that the categorical noun is pointing to a previously mentioned idea. See the excerpt from Bugg (2013, p. 1158) in Box 5.7. Notice how the underlined categorical nouns in the second sentence substitute for the more specific idea expressed in the first sentence.

BOX 5.6. Repetition through Pronoun Use

The temple, proposed for an overwhelmingly Anglo-Australian rural–residential area made up of mega homes and hobby farms, was denied planning permission by local government planners. It also encountered significant opposition from the local community. Drawing upon interviews with local planners, residents and members of the Hindu temple congregation, as well as analysis of policy documentation, this article examines the negotiation of citizenship and belonging at the local scale through the disruption of an elite, Anglo-Australian landscape.

BOX 5.7. Repetition through the Use of Categorical Nouns

The narratives presented by local residents in both letters of submission to local government and in interviews reflect particular understandings of rural space and of themselves in relation to family, neighbours and more broadly the Australian nation. These perceptions and experiences of rural–urban fringe space have important implications for the exclusion or inclusion of non-white groups.

ELLIPSIS

Ellipsis occurs when the key word or idea is dropped but some nonspecific reminder of its existence is included. Notice how the word *another* is used to refer to *letter* in the excerpt from Bugg (2013, p. 1161) in Box 5.8.

ELABORATION

Elaboration occurs when a more specific word or idea is substituted for the key word or idea. This might be achieved through something like the selection of a more specific or concrete word or through the creation of an expanded noun phrase, as we discussed in Chapter 4. Notice how the general concept of multiculturalism is replaced by a noun phrase with the same meaning in the excerpt from Bugg (2013, p. 1152) in Box 5.9.

Repetition through substitution is a primary cohesive strategy accomplished through many different cohesive devices in academic writing. The use of repetition through substitution is required to fulfill the expectations of the reader. Try your hand at identifying and explaining the cohesive devices used to substitute for key words and ideas in the excerpt from Walker-Williams et al. (2012, p. 621) in Practice Exercise 5.5. You can check your answers in the Appendix.

BOX 5.8. Repetition through Ellipsis

One letter to Council from the Swaminarayans noted, "Rural land is preferable for a temple. We need the site in a peaceful and rural area" (Letter of submission 2009). Another argued: "The land itself is in a peaceful and calm area, so it will be good for our worship and our practices. It is important for worshippers to have a silent and peaceful environment for prayers."

BOX 5.9. Repetition through Elaboration

Despite explicit government direction to facilitate and implement multicultural planning, policy and service frameworks, local government attempts to embrace multiculturalism in the built environment could best be described as ad hoc (Sandercock and Kliger 1998). Although many local governments have implemented multicultural arts and food festivals, studies show that they are often "reluctant to participate in culturally inclusive practices" (Thompson 2003:278).

PRACTICE EXERCISE 5.5. Identifying Cohesive Devices Used for Repetition

1. Identify all instances of exact repetition and repetition through substitution.
2. For each instance you identify, explain exactly what cohesive device is used to achieve the repetition.

From the prevalence results for constructive coping, posttraumatic growth and psychological well-being it was seen that more than half of the women manifested constructive coping, while only 42% of the participants manifested coping self-efficacy. This seems to be a discrepancy but the explanation may lie in the low self-esteem manifested by these women. Only 45% obtained high self-esteem scores and this corresponds with the 42% who scored high on coping self-efficacy. These findings clearly indicate the harm that was done to essential self-related strengths in these women and is supported by the work of Saffy (2003). Of the participants, two thirds manifested posttraumatic growth, which is higher than levels of posttraumatic growth seen in previous studies (Peltzer, 2000).

Reader Cues

Reader cues are another category of cohesive devices. Reader cues are words or phrases that writers use that essentially tell the reader what the writer wants them to do. Reader cues indicate how the writer wants the reader to follow the writer's thought progression. Reader cues can indicate how a writer wants the reader to understand ideas. For example, the use of *because* indicates that the writer wants the reader to understand the ideas presented as having a cause–effect relationship. Reader cues can also be used by the writer to direct readers' attention so that readers follow arguments in the way that the writer wishes. For instance, the use of a phrase like *as we have mentioned* indicates that the writer is directing readers to remember that the subsequent idea has already been discussed, so whatever has been previously established about this idea in the writer's text should be applied in understanding whatever new information is given. Reader cues are similar to metacommentary in the sense that they direct the readers' interpretation and understanding of the text. At times, the difference between reader cues and metacommentary may be indistinguishable.

Reader cues are very common in academic writing. Although these cues can be used to create cohesion at the macro- and meso-levels, these cues primarily function at the micro-level. Some reader cues can be used to link ideas within sentences, and some link ideas between sentences within paragraphs. We discuss three types of cohesive devices used as reader cues: conjunctions, transitions, and directional cues.

Conjunctions

Conjunctions are used to connect ideas within sentences. Writers use conjunctions to cue readers to understand the relationship between ideas in specific ways. There are different types of conjunctions: coordinating, subordinating, and correlative. It isn't all that important that you know the exact differences between the types, but it is important that you use conjunctions in your writing. Conjunctions help writers to cue readers that relationships between ideas like the following are occurring: addition, choice, reason, concession, condition, time, comparison, contrast. They also help writers to express time and manner relationships. See Table 5.5 for a sample list of conjunctions and the relationships they express. This list is far from exhaustive. As always, we recommend Googling to find more complete lists and to see examples. One list that we particularly like can be found at *www.smart-words.org/linking-words/conjunctions.html.*

Conjunctions not only help writers guide readers to understanding the relationship between ideas, but they also allow writers to add information to their sentences. Academic writing, as we have mentioned, is dense. Each sentence needs to carry as much information as it possibly can without creating confusion. But academic writing is also concise. Sentences carry a lot of information so that there don't have to be as many sentences. Conjunctions

TABLE 5.5. Conjunctions and Their Functions			
Functions	**Coordinating**	**Subordinating**	**Correlative**
Addition	*and*		
Choice	*or, nor*		
Reason	*for, so*	*because, so that*	
Comparison		*than, rather than*	
Contrast	*but, yet*	*whereas, while, despite*	
Concession		*although, even though, while*	
Condition		*if, unless, even if, provided that*	
Time		*before, after, since, until, when, once*	
Manner		*as if, as though*	
Equality			*both . . . and* *neither . . . nor* *not only . . . but* *whether . . . or* *either . . . or*

allow writers to create cohesion between multiple ideas within sentences so that they can write fewer sentences. See the excerpt from Hawkins et al. (2014, p. 342) in Table 5.6 and the commentary for a discussion of how conjunctions are used to create cohesion within a sentence and how they contribute to the creation of dense sentences.

Transitions

Transition words and phrases are used to link ideas between sentences. They express many of the same relationships that conjunctions express, such as addition and contrast, among others, but they express those relationships between rather than within sentences. (However, it is also true that transitions are sometimes used within sentences.) In addition, transitions are used for some functions that are not as common for conjunctions, such as summary, generalization, emphasis, conclusion, and exemplification. New writers generally notice and use transitions, but they actually sometimes overuse transitions. In academic writing, transitions are important for cohesion, but many of the cohesive devices used for repetition are more common. See Table 5.7 for a sample list of transitions and the relationships they express. As always, we recommend Googling to find more complete lists and to see examples.

See the excerpt from Singh and McKleroy (2011, p. 35) in Table 5.8 and the commentary for a discussion of how conjunctions and transitions create cohesion within and between sentences.

TABLE 5.6. Conjunctions for Cohesion and Density of Prose
Text
As critical geographers, we aim to convey how these positions of power, authority and prestige are socially constructed, profoundly oppressive and not inevitable so that more graduate students start questioning, criticizing and resisting the reproduction of such unequal power relations within academia.
Commentary
The text contains 42 words, which in everyday personal writing would be considered far too long, but it is fairly normal for academic writing. As you can see, the sentence carries multiple ideas—between two and four. The authors appear to want to convey three ideas about how certain positions are (1) constructed, (2) oppressive, and (3) not inevitable. It is possible that the authors will discuss all of these as one idea, or the authors could be planning to discuss each idea separately. The conjunction *so that* is used to indicate that the reason those three ideas are addressed is to achieve (4) graduate students' questioning, criticizing, and resisting. Thus the conjunction allows the authors to express more than one idea in the sentence, and it simultaneously allows them to propose a relationship between those ideas.

TABLE 5.7. Transitions and Their Functions	
Functions	**Transitions**
Addition	*moreover, furthermore, in addition*
Choice	*instead, on the other hand*
Reason	*therefore, thus, as a result, consequently, for this reason*
Comparison	*similarly, likewise, like*
Contrast	*however, in contrast, unlike, rather, regardless*
Concession	*nevertheless, nonetheless, granted, of course, given that, granted that, considering that*
Equality	*equally important*
Emphasis	*in fact, indeed, notably, in particular, namely, above all*
Generalization/Summary/Conclusion	*in general, generally, usually, in sum, to summarize, in conclusion, to conclude, finally*
Exemplification	*for example, for instance, to illustrate*

Directional Cues

Writers' and readers' relationships with written texts are not spatial; that is, they do not locate things in the text in relation to their own bodies the way they might in a physical space. For example, when a person is in a room, and you ask the person where something is, he will tell you where it is in relation to another object, your body, or his body. Written texts do not have this kind of physical space, but they do have a kind of imagined space that both writers and readers understand. The space of written text may be measured in two ways: sequentially, as in before and after, or vertically, as in above and below. It is generally preferred to think of the space of academic texts sequentially. Because writers are trying to guide their readers through a problem–conclusion argument and the argument invariably includes cause–effect, writers will from time to time need to spatially orient their readers. In particular, writers will need to metaphorically ask readers to remember something that writers don't want to repeat.

These types of spatial reminders are important for maintaining the flow of the argument as they acknowledge the important fact that readers expect writers to make it easy for them to follow the argument. Readers need writers to remind them of what they should be thinking about, because it is not the readers' job in academic writing to "bring it all together"; it is the writers' job. Also, writers need to anticipate that at certain points, readers may want information that writers plan to provide at a later point, so writers can orient readers to this plan as a way to address readers' potential objections. Spatial reminders include phrases such as the following: *as mentioned earlier, as previously discussed, the aforementioned . . . , the former, as follows, following, the latter,* and *later.* You may also see writers use words such as *above* or *below* when referring to information, but this may not be acceptable in all disciplines.

Grammar

In addition to cohesive devices that primarily rely on the use of words or phrases such as those used for repetition and reader cues, there are some grammatical constructions that can also create cohesion. These constructions function in much the same way that the word- and phrase-based cohesive devices do; they link ideas within and between sentences. In so doing, they facilitate the imagined interactions between writers and readers by adding clarity and providing writers with more ways to add information to their sentences and paragraphs. There are two uses of grammar that we find particularly useful for cohesion: parallel structure and a blending of active and passive voice.

TABLE 5.8. Conjunctions and Transitions for Cohesion and Density of Prose
Text
[1]**Although** a thorough review of the identity development scholarship with regard to race/ethnicity and gender identity development is beyond the scope of this article, it is important to discuss these models briefly. [2]Racial/ethnic identity development models share a perspective that people of color move from an unawareness of oppression to recognizing a specific experience of racism. [3]**Then**, they may align with people of their own race/ethnicity **before** moving to a more integrated view of their race/ethnicity (Helms, 1989; Ibrahim, Ohnishi, & Sandhu, 1997; Rockquemore, Brunsma, & Delgado, 2009). [4]**Similarly**, transgender identity development models follow a process where individuals develop awareness of one's self as differently gendered from one's assigned biological sex, finding information and support, exploring one's identity, and synthesizing a transgender identity (Lev, 2004; Morgan & Stevens, 2008).
Commentary
As we have discussed, conjunctions allow writers to include more ideas in their sentences and to propose relationships between those ideas. *Although* in sentence 1 has this function. It enables the authors to express two ideas and acknowledge that these ideas stand in contrast to one another. Sentence 2 expresses only one idea, the first step in a process. *Then* in sentence 3 functions as a transition of time, indicating that the next step of the process presented in sentence 2 is given in sentence 3. *Before* in sentence 3 functions as a conjunction of time and helps the authors to indicate what the next step in the process would be. *Similarly* functions as a transition, helping the authors to introduce a different process that follows a similar pattern. Through the use of conjunctions and transitions the authors are able to effectively guide readers through six different pieces of information and their relationships to one another in only four sentences.

Parallel Structure

We discussed the concept of parallelism as a structural consideration in Chapter 4. However, parallel structure is also a cohesive device because it can help readers to see connections between ideas. As you may recall, parallel structure refers to using the same grammatical pattern to express ideas that are equal, and it is also related to addressing topics in the same order in which you introduced them. The basic point of parallel structure is that if a writer proposes a pattern, the reader expects the writer to follow the pattern. When writers do not follow the patterns they propose, readers invariably become confused and have trouble following the argument. Parallel structure can be used at all levels, and we discussed some of those uses in Chapter 4. In this section, we focus on how parallel structure can be used to create cohesion between paragraphs within a section.

Let's consider for a moment the classification organizational pattern. When writers classify, they break a topic into smaller parts. If the classification is not hierarchical, all of the parts are considered equal. If a writer plans to discuss each part of the classification separately, perhaps in separate paragraphs, the writer can use parallel structure to link the paragraphs. Parallel structure in this case would mean that every paragraph essentially begins the same way (i.e., a similar sentence pattern), includes the same type of information in the same order, and uses very similar sentence types at the same places in each paragraph. In Box 5.10, notice how Singh and McKleroy (2011, pp. 40–41) establish a pattern for discussing each of their themes in the first paragraph of their discussion and follow this pattern in each of the following five paragraphs.

Blending of Active and Passive Voice

Active voice is used when the subject of the sentence performs the action (e.g., "I wrote the essay"). Passive voice is used when the subject of the sentence receives the action of the verb (e.g., "The essay was written by me"). Most academic writers will tell you how important it is to use the active voice, and it is. However, blending your use of the active and passive voices can be a cohesive device. Do you remember the repeat-old-information-add-new-information pattern that we mentioned at the beginning of this chapter? Well, blending the active and passive voices can facilitate the use of this pattern. Take a look at the excerpt from Bugg (2013, pp. 1159–1160) in Table 5.9 and the commentary that accompanies it.

The ways in which grammar is used as a cohesive device are certainly more subtle than either repetition or reader cues, and it is likely that readers respond to grammar use more or less unconsciously. However, learning to use parallel structure and to blend the active and passive voices can add a level of sophistication to your writing that your readers will appreciate.

BOX 5.10. Parallel Structure as a Cohesive Device at the Meso-Level

Paragraph 1

Similar to previous studies of the resilience and coping of LGBTQ persons (Gonzalez, 2008; Lewis, 2008; Singh, Hays, & Watson, in press), the participants in this study described the pride they developed in *both* their racial/ethnic and gender identities as integral to their resilience to traumatic life events.

Paragraph 2

The finding that navigating family relationships was a key aspect of both their resilience and trauma experiences is also congruent with previous literature with LGB people of color (Burnes, 2006; Chan, 1989; Singh et al., 2006).

Paragraph 3

In addition to family support, having access to financial and medical resources supported participants' resilience to traumatic life experiences. Similar to previous studies (Lewis, 2008; Nemoto et al., 2004), participants described difficulty "passing" in their gender identity when they did not have access to medical care and/or could not afford treatment.

Paragraph 4

The finding that participants' resilience entailed connecting with an activist transgender people of color community is similar to previous studies of transgender persons' resilience (Gonzalez, 2008; Singh, et al., in press) and the coping resources of LGBQ persons of color (Chan, 1989; Singh et al., 2006).

Paragraph 5

Finally, the finding that participants accessed their spirituality as a source of resilience—which then led to increased hope about their future as transgender people of color—is similar to other qualitative investigations of racial/ethnic minorities who have survived traumatic life events (Singh, 2006; Stevens, 1997).

TABLE 5.9. Blending Active and Passive Voice as a Cohesive Device

Text

[1]Graham <u>asserts</u> that heritage "does not engage with the study of the past. [2]Instead, it **is concerned** with the ways in which selective material artefacts, mythologies, memories and traditions <u>become</u> resources for the present" (Graham 2002:1004). [3]In the Hindu temple case study, local residents <u>celebrate</u> specific histories (the landed English gentleman and colonial settler) and <u>exclude</u> others (Indigenous and migrant histories). [4]Residents <u>appeal</u> to Australia's British colonial heritage while simultaneously bypassing its history of contemporary multiculturalism (Leung 2008). [5]This has been a frequent tactic in the creation of white space in Australia with the erasure of Indigenous history (Shaw 2006). [6]The rural **is perceived** as a place of traditional or authentic "Australianness", where homes built in the style of English manors <u>evoke</u> the landed gentry and upper classes (Bressey 2009).

Commentary

The active verbs have been underlined, and the passive verbs are in bold. As you can see, there are clearly more active verbs, which is the way that it should be. However, the passive verbs are facilitating flow in this paragraph. In sentence 1, the author introduces the concept of *heritage*. In sentence 1, *heritage* functions as the subject of the noun clause and performs the action *does not engage*. However, the point of the paragraph is not to focus on something heritage does but rather how heritage is acted upon by others. Accordingly, sentence 2 shifts *heritage,* which is replaced by the pronoun *it,* to an object role by using the passive construction *is concerned*. The author had to do this for probably two reasons. One reason is that the meaning of *heritage* limits the number of actions it could possibly perform, so perhaps using it in the active voice again would not have made sense. Another reason is that trying to stay in the active voice and compose a sentence that expressed the same idea as sentence 2 would have required the author to come up with a person who said this about *heritage*, and perhaps no one said it—it is just a general idea. In any case, the person who said it really is not important, so the passive voice allows the author to leave the subject out. Sentence 6 also uses the passive voice. In the sentences prior, the author has established that *residents* in the case study glorify the colonial history of Australia, which means that they downplay the indigenous history. In sentence 6, the author no longer wishes to talk about what the residents do, she wants to discuss the results of their actions—how the concept of the *rural* has been acted upon by others. She uses the passive voice to shift the focus from the residents to the results (i.e., how the rural is perceived). Thus, as a cohesive device, blending the active and passive voices allows the author to omit unnecessary subjects (e.g., the case of heritage) and appear more neutral by not including any subjects that "do" anything negative, even though there is something that she considers to be a negative result (e.g., the case of *rural*).

We suggest that you spend some time noticing and appreciating the ways that grammar guides you as a reader. We also suggest that you notice when grammar creates an obstacle for you as a reader. By noticing when it helps and when it doesn't, you will hopefully gain a deeper understanding of how you can use grammar to improve your cohesion.

In order to pull everything together from this chapter and apply it, review some of your own writing using the instructions in Practice Exercise 5.6.

PRACTICE EXERCISE 5.6. Reviewing Your Own Writing

1. Select a multiparagraph section of any paper that you may have written.
2. Look for examples of hedging. Are you hedging enough? Are you using a variety of hedging devices?
3. Look for examples of signal phrases and signal verbs. In your writing, are shifts between your voice and the voices of those you are integrating into your writing clear? If not, how can you clarify those shifts? When you use signal verbs, are the verbs you have chosen accurately reflecting the attitudes of the other voices you are integrating?
4. Look for examples of metacommentary. Is your use of metacommentary helpful to aligning the reader's understanding of your argument with your own? If you didn't use any metacommentary, would your argument be clearer or more persuasive if you did?
5. Look for examples of meso-level cohesion (i.e., cohesion between paragraphs). Would a reader clearly understand how the ideas you are expressing in different paragraphs are connected?
6. Look for examples of micro-level cohesion (i.e., cohesion between ideas within sentences and cohesion between sentences). You should be using a wide variety of cohesive strategies. Which strategies are you using most often? Which strategies are you not using? How could you improve your micro-level cohesion?

CHAPTER SUMMARY AND REMINDERS

As we have said in this chapter, we want you to gain a deeper understanding of how academic writing language is influenced by writer–reader roles. We hope that you have gotten some ideas for steps that you can take to develop your ability to write using a rational tone and cohesive style. See Summary Table 5.1 for a reminder list of awareness and action suggestions from this chapter.

SUMMARY TABLE 5.1. AWARENESS AND ACTION REMINDERS

Be aware . . .	Take action . . .
Academic writers need to use a rational tone, which means that they should adopt an attitude that is neutral, impersonal, and reasonable.	Identify and notice the ways that hedging, signal phrases, and metacommentary are used in your discipline's writing, and begin using them in your own writing.
Hedging, signal phrases, and metacommentary contribute to a rational tone.	Use the Internet to expand your repertoire of writing language words.
Cohesive devices are used at the macro-, meso-, and micro-levels to establish links between ideas that will allow the reader to follow the writer's argument easily.	Repeat often in a variety of ways.
Writers can use repetition, reader cues, and grammar to create cohesion.	Tell your readers what you want them to think and where you want them to go in your text using cohesive devices.
Repetition is by far the most used and most important strategy for creating cohesion.	Create and follow patterns in your writing to help your argument flow more smoothly.

CHAPTER 6

Coaching Yourself to Completion

In Chapters 4 and 5, we focused on the product of academic writing (i.e., the written text). We discussed the communication and language skills that are actually used to compose that product. However, academic writing is more than a product, it is also a process. Understanding how to navigate that process is a skill that is just as important as any of the skills involved in actually composing the product. We imagine that you have already participated in the academic writing process, so you probably already know that the writing process can be complex, confusing, messy, frustrating, stressful, and tiring. And the process can be all of these things *before* you ever actually put your fingers on the keyboard to write your text. For us, the key to navigating this process is understanding how to coach yourself through the process.

In this chapter, we discuss how personal considerations such as deeply embedded preferences, past experiences, and current feelings may influence your participation in the academic writing process. We share strategies and ideas that we hope will help you to manage your participation in the writing process in ways that work for you. Our **awareness focus** for this chapter is to help you to develop an understanding of the personal considerations that may have an impact on your participation in the academic writing process. Our **action focus** includes suggestions and strategies you can use to coach yourself through the entire writing process.

SELF-COACHING AND THE WRITING PROCESS

In sports, coaches understand that coaching a single event (e.g., game or match) is something more than just showing up and coaching at that event. They generally understand an event as having three phases that require coaching—a preplaying phase, a while-playing phase, and a postplaying phase. Their duties and responsibilities as coaches shift according to the phase. Likewise, we think that one of things that you should understand in your self-coaching role is that the writing process has three distinct phases—a prewriting phase, a while-writing phase, and a postwriting phase—and that each phase is potentially influenced by a variety of personal considerations that may affect your ability to write. The techniques you adopt for coaching yourself in each phase will naturally vary according to the phase of the writing process in which you find yourself and the specific consideration(s) that affect you.

In general, we believe that your general approach to self-coaching at any phase of the writing process should be positive and strengths-based. A classic rule in positive, strengths-based coaching is to focus on people's strengths and to coach them to use these strengths to overcome their growing edges. (Growing edges are those places where you can improve.) In self-coaching, this means that, rather than trying to force yourself to immediately become someone you are not in order to achieve a goal, you try to understand how to use the strengths you already have to achieve your goals.

For instance, let's imagine a fairly typical situation wherein a person has the goal of being a successful, published academic writer. Of course, this person naturally wants to take advantage of all opportunities that she has to work on writing projects that lead to publication in her discipline. However, let's imagine that one of this person's growing edges is overcommitment. She finds it hard to say no to any writing project. This means that she is frequently juggling multiple writing projects with multiple collaborators at the same time. This growing edge could lead to disaster if she is unable to follow through on her commitments, but if she accesses and uses some of her strengths, she may be able to avoid disaster and meet her commitments.

Let's imagine that one of this person's strengths includes having a very realistic sense of how long it will take her to write different texts. Another of her strengths is that she is very disciplined about creating and following to-do lists. This person can use her realistic sense of how long it will take her to write a text to create to-do lists that are realistic and accurate for the time frame available. Then she can use her self-discipline for following these realistic and accurate to-do lists to prioritize her multiple commitments so that even though she is overcommitted, she can still meet her multiple commitments. So, in the end, this person's realistic sense of time and her ability to create and follow a plan will compensate for her overcommitment provided that she uses her strengths properly. This person's growing edge of overcommitting will not necessarily be resolved, but it will not be an obstacle that negatively affects her participation in the academic writing process. (As a longer term solution, we would also advise this person to also explore why she overcommits and to consider her own willingness to change that pattern.)

Of course, before you can leverage your strengths to overcome your growing edges, you do have to have some awareness of what your strengths and growing edges are. So one of the actions we suggest now and throughout this chapter is fiercely honest self-reflection. This type of self-reflection is not the kind by which you provide answers based on your best day or your worst day or what you wish were true. Rather, your answers are based on what is real and true for you on a daily and consistent basis. Good self-coaching for your academic writing journey depends in large part upon your willingness and desire to know and accept yourself. You have to work with the "you" that is presently available, not that other you that has not arrived yet. You can work on transforming some of your growing edges to new strengths as you continue your academic writing journey, but until you have developed those new strengths, you will need to use the strengths you currently have to overcome the growing edges that you currently have.

We would like you to begin your self-coaching by simply reflecting on your strengths and challenges with regard to academic writing in Practice Exercise 6.1.

PRACTICE EXERCISE 6.1. Self-Reflection for Positive, Strengths-Based Self-Coaching

Take a moment to answer the following questions and consider all three phases of the writing process (i.e., prewriting, while-writing, and postwriting) as you answer:

- What are the most common challenges you face in your academic writing process?
- What are your strengths when it comes to your academic writing process?
- How might you use your strengths to help address the growing edges you have in your academic writing process?

GOAL SETTING AND THE WRITING PROCESS

Once you have identified your strengths and growing edges, you are in a better position to coach yourself through the three phases of the writing process. One of the coaching skills that you will need in all three phases is the ability to set goals. There are seven hallmarks for coaching yourself to set good goals that you can actually meet:

1. Goals should be positive.
2. Goals should be specific.

3. Goals anticipate challenges.
4. Goals should be achievable and reassessed.
5. Goals should be a mix of short-term and long-term objectives.
6. Goals should be shared.
7. Goal making should be rewarded.

So how does all of this apply to setting goals as an academic writer? First of all, your writing goals should be framed positively. When you say that your writing goal is "not to procrastinate," then your brain literally hears "procrastinate," and you tend to immediately have negative feelings. Instead, place your goal in the positive—and we are not talking about some la-la land where there are rainbows and unicorns. We are talking about positive reality: "My goal is to increase my writing" or "My goal is to write more often." Your thoughts literally shift into "Oh, yeah. I can do that." And that is the type of thinking that enhances motivation and goal completion.

Once you have a goal that is written in a positive tone, then the challenge is to make it specific. Saying you want to write regularly is a great start, but you need to back up that great start with a "how to do that" type of specificity. For instance, under the larger goal of wanting to increase your writing, you could say, "My goal is to write for an hour three times a week." Boom. You nailed it. This writing goal is not only positive, but it is specific and guides you exactly in the direction of becoming a more regular writer.

In addition to being specific, your writing goals should anticipate challenges. This is an essential step, as we can set goals all day that are positive and specific—but if we do not anticipate the challenges we will face in meeting these writing goals, then (you guessed it) we will tend not to meet our goals. Let's stay with the example of wanting to increase your writing. What would be the challenges currently in your life in doing this? Is it your family, job, workload, or recreation time that immediately feels like the challenge? Identifying the challenges, whatever they are, and then identifying a "work-around" in which you address that challenge in advance will set you up to successfully meet your writing goals. If you are a better writer at night but you have to get up early for your job, then you have to identify how to work around that challenge. Maybe you could start your hour of writing 1 hour earlier in the evening—which might mean eating dinner 1 hour earlier, too, which might mean the need to discuss this goal and your need for support with this goal with your family or roommates if you have a communal dinner. You get the idea. Knowing what the challenges are going to be in meeting your goal will give you smooth sailing over those obstacles every time.

Now that you have anticipated the obstacles to your writing goals, then you can assess whether your goal is actually achievable. This is typically a step in goal setting that you do often—asking yourself, "Is this a good goal that I can realistically meet?" We have worked with plenty of students who were binge writers who wanted their goal to be writing every day. Well, that is a big jump from being a binge writer, but there are definitely some goals that are more realistic to help with that transition to increasing their writing. For instance, for a binge writer, setting a goal of writing for two 3-hour blocks in a week might be a more realistic and achievable goal than writing for an hour each day. It is crucial to reassess goals, so if this was your goal and you did not achieve it, it is important to ask, "What would make this a better goal that I can achieve?" It could be something as simple as changing the "where" of the goal, such as staying late at work to write or writing at a coffeehouse, or the issue could be larger and actually have to do with the content of what you did with your writing blocks (e.g., checked social media the entire time) or the increments of time set (e.g., wrote for 1 hour instead of 3). Reassessing your goals often and early helps keep you on track for your larger goals of improving your academic writing.

Next, make sure to ask yourself what your short-term and long-term goals are. They are both important, and also very different. For example, you may have a short-term goal to complete a paper for a class, but a long-term goal is to turn that paper into something that is publishable in your field. You would need to identify short-term goals to finish your paper (e.g., 1 day writing at a coffeehouse) versus the long-term goal of publishing your paper (e.g., answering *when, where,* and *how* questions, including questions of whether you will have a collaborator and how you will integrate professors' feedback). Consistently setting short-term and long-term goals can help keep you out of a writing rut as well. We work with plenty of students who move from paper to paper writing assignments in the short term, such as a semester, but then do not connect these paper writing assignments to their overall goal (e.g., graduation!). It can really increase motivation if you know how mini-writing goals fit into your overall long-term goals for your life.

Another very common aspect of goal setting is sharing the goals with others you trust, as this creates accountability for meeting your goals. This could be as formal as participating in a writing group regularly or as informal as talking over your upcoming goals with a peer, partner, or family member. We have seen students create Facebook groups and use other types of social media and texting platforms to create goal-sharing accountability, where people post from daily to weekly on their goal setting. No matter how you set up your goal sharing—whether it is with one or lots of people—we are often more accountable to meeting our writing goals when we speak them out loud to someone else. Even better is sharing your goals and then following up with those with whom you have shared your goals to report your progress, from the deep lows to the soaring highs and everything in between, in meeting your academic writing goals.

The last, and perhaps most important, aspect of goal setting in academic writing is planning rewards for meeting your goals. Meeting your writing goals is a big deal, and we believe you should celebrate yourself accordingly. Rewards, as we know in psychology, positively reinforce accomplishments, thus increasing motivation and success. Sometimes, we see students mistake what we mean by rewards. Rewards can be small, medium, or large and should make our lives more enjoyable, rather than less enjoyable. For instance, when you complete that annotated bibliography for class, reward yourself with a long, hot bath or binge watching the favorite television show that you fell behind on because you were writing. Save the big rewards—dinners and outings with loved ones—for the big writing goal completions, so that they are truly special and something you can look forward to while you are working hard on your writing goals. Regardless, do not skip your rewards! Even if it is a simple reward, do it— because rewards help you meet your next writing goals. Explore your current goal-setting abilities by completing Practice Exercise 6.2.

PRACTICE EXERCISE 6.2. Goal Setting as a Self-Coaching Skill

Identify three goals to improve your academic writing process. Then run the three goals through the following questions to see what needs to be tweaked:

- Is your goal written using positive language?
- Is your goal specific?
- Does your goal anticipate challenges?
- Is your goal achievable and easy to reassess?
- Does your goal have short-term and long-term objectives?
- Who could you share your goal with in order to be accountable to your goals?
- How will you reward yourself for meeting your goal?

PERSONAL CONSIDERATIONS AND THE WRITING PROCESS

Understanding how to set goals that you can actually meet is an important first step in the writing process, and the second step is coaching yourself to follow through on meeting those goals. Good self-coaching includes understanding yourself and the impact that your deeply embedded personal preferences, past experiences, and current feelings may have on your ability to follow through on meeting your goals. Some of the personal considerations that may affect you include your personal time/space orientation and your personal coping styles, which we consider to be deeply embedded personal preferences. Other personal considerations that may affect you include your personal motivation, which is related to your current feelings, and the voices in your head, which are related to your past experiences.

Personal Time/Space Orientation

We think of your personal time/space orientation as the deeply embedded personal preferences you have toward time and space. You could think of the possible preferences as a continuum. At one end of the continuum the descriptor might be "very structured," and at the other end, "very free flowing." If you are more in the direction of the "very structured" end, you are probably a person who does what they are supposed to do when they are supposed to do it. You are probably a person who likes to plan and schedule. You are probably a person who appreciates orderliness and organization. You are probably also the kind of person who cares about knowing and following the rules.

If you are more in the direction of the "very free flowing" end, you are probably a person who has a more flexible or spontaneous view of time and space. You are probably a person who likes to wait and see what happens or go with the flow. You may also be the kind of person who only cares about knowing the rules so that you can judge when you want to follow them and when you don't (i.e., you view rules as suggestions rather than mandates).

You may already have a clear idea of which time/space orientation you have, but just in case you haven't figured that out yet, answer the following questions:

- You have a "free" day, and you get to decide what you want to do with your day! Do you prefer to make plans to see people and have a schedule for the day, or do you prefer to keep your day flexible and see how the day goes?
- Think about your bank account. Do you know exactly how much money you have in your account, or do you just have a general idea of whether there is enough or not enough money in your account?

Both time/space orientations have their strengths and growing edges with respect to academic writing. The person who has a more structured time/space orientation will likely do well with the aspects of academic writing that require planning and following rules or formulas, whereas the person with a more free-flowing time/space orientation may struggle with these aspects. The highly structured aspects of academic writing will probably appeal to the person with the more structured time/space orientation. However, this person may struggle with some of the messier tasks involved in academic writing, such as brainstorming, wide-angle research, and synthesizing information from lots of different sources. On the other hand, the person with a more free-flowing orientation will likely enjoy the freedom and flexibility offered by these tasks to the rules and structures required by other tasks.

Although both the more structured and the more free-flowing time/space orientations have strengths, it is true that people with a more structured time/space orientation have perhaps a natural advantage with specific aspects of the academic writing process. For example, they are likely to be more willing and more practiced with managing time, planning, and following a plan. They may have a more realistic sense of the time required to complete tasks due to their more structured sense of time. They are likely to be motivated to meet deadlines, and they will prefer working according to an organized plan. People with a more free-flowing time/space orientation will likely struggle with these time management and planning aspects, which are both very important in the academic writing process, so they will need to assess how their strengths can be leveraged to overcome their growing edges.

For those with a more structured time/space orientation, we recommend the following three strategies for leveraging your structure-based strengths: Use a deadline approach to writing, become a regular writer, and identify the best places for productive writing.

1. *Use a deadline approach to writing.* Those of you with a more structured time/space orientation are inherently motivated by deadlines. They help you to organize time and space, so you may view them with some degree of positivity. At the very least, you have a strong respect for deadlines, and you have a strong desire to meet them. That's great! There are lots of deadlines in the academic writing process, and your willingness and desire to meet them will be greatly appreciated by your readers. The deadline approach that we recommend is a simple scheduling technique that comprises the following steps:

- Make a list of the things you need to do in order to finish your written text.
- Next to each item, record the amount of time you think it will take. (Be realistic to the point of being cautious in these predictions.)
- Add up the total time it will take to complete all items in the list. Then, add 5 extra hours just because anything could happen.
- Take out your calendar (on your phone, in your planner, etc.).
- Find the ultimate deadline. Factoring in the total number of hours you have estimated, work backward and schedule writing appointments for yourself. Obviously, you will not have the same amount of time each day, so schedule the amount of time for each appointment according to what you expect the demands of those days to be. Do not wait until the day of the appointment to decide how much time you have. The key is to actually create writing appointments just as you would a doctor's appointment and to work your life around those appointments rather than those appointments around your life.
- As you schedule your writing appointments, identify the specific space in which you intend to work for that appointment (e.g., one appointment could be in your dining room, another could be in your favorite coffee shop).
- Share your calendar with your writing appointments with those

whose schedules may be affected by your schedule. Let them know that these appointments are important to you and your ability to finish your writing on time. Enlist the cooperation of family and friends to help you work around these appointments just as you would if you had a dentist appointment.

2. *Become a regular writer.* Many students—and faculty members too—tell themselves they do not have time to write. This can be a typical response, because often we have learned that "writing" always means putting pen to paper or words on an electronic document. For people who have a more structured time/space orientation, it will likely work best to find times in your schedule to write regularly a certain number of days of the week, even when you may not have a close deadline or a specific writing task, whether you set a regular time (e.g., early morning before the kids get up or late night when you are home from classes) or identify captured time between classes as your writing/thinking time. During these regular sessions, anything you are doing that goes into past, current, or future writing counts. That means anything—from responding to feedback, searching for relevant literature, outlining, reading, thinking about how you will build your argument, discussing your topic with peers or faculty, and even learning how to use a program or other tool that you will eventually need to understand and use for your writing.

3. *Identify the best places for you to write.* In the many years we have taught academic writing, we have heard all sorts of stories about where people like to write—from sitting on couches with a laptop (not always the best ergonomically, of course) and working on a desktop computer to writing in a coffee shop or other public venue. If you have a more structured time/space orientation, the space in which you work is likely an important part of your process. You may want to claim a place in your home and set it up so that it is always ready for you. You may want to establish certain rituals about your use of that space, such as tidying it up when you finish so that it is ready for you to begin again or creating a sense of relaxation by lighting a candle when you sit down to write and blowing it out when you finish. You might also consider wrapping up your writing sessions by using the electronic post-it function on your computer to create a note that will appear on your screen that lets you know what you need to work on the next time you sit down to write. If there is no space in your home that works for you, we suggest that you look at places such as public and/or university libraries—it does not have to be your own university in order for you to use the library. You can usually find a quiet space that is consistently unoccupied that you can claim as your own. If your space is not at home, you will want to be sure that you have everything you need to create the structured atmosphere that you prefer. This will probably entail having a dedicated writing kit of some kind, perhaps a bag that is always prepared with the things that you need while you write. Again, the rituals of how you set up and break down your public writing space can be very useful

for helping you to shift to and from your academic writer identity to your other identities.

The natural strengths of a person with a more structured time/space orientation ensure that the time management aspect of the writing process will be more manageable for him. It does not mean that he will never struggle with deadlines or have to engage in binge writing, because everyone does at some point. However, writers with a more structured time/space orientation may struggle with what we have called the messier aspects of writing—those tasks that are more open-ended or ambiguous. For example, good writing requires a great deal of rereading and rewriting during the writing process. A good writer frequently rereads what he has written to ensure that his argument is coherently organized and cohesively expressed. This frequent rereading results in many changes, big and small, en route to finishing a writing project. If you don't believe us, take a look at the article at *www.theatlantic.com/entertainment/archive/2013/01/my-pencils-outlast-their-erasers-great-writers-on-the-art-of-revision/267011*, which includes the thoughts of 20 famous authors on rewriting. This brings us to one skill that people with more structured time/space orientations may want to develop: Be willing to allow your plan to change.

4. *Be willing to allow your plan to change.* As we have said, revision is a natural part of the writing process, and you will revise continuously as you write. A large part of finishing your writing is also knowing when you are headed in a successful direction in your academic writing and when you need to switch course. For instance, sometimes you will be following a certain line of reasoning, but you may discover while writing that new literature doesn't fit in with that line of reasoning, or you may realize as you write (remember the idea of writing to learn) that the way you had understood something has changed as you write and the change somehow affects your line of reasoning. Do you keep going, or do you head down another path?

As a deadline-motivated person, you will probably want to keep going and to try to "make it work." However, we suggest that you at least consider speaking with peers or professors, searching the literature again, or using mind maps and other brainstorming tools to revisit your line of reasoning. If you try one of these strategies and find a way to maintain your line of reasoning, go for it. On the other hand, if you fundamentally realize that your line of reasoning is not working, you need to change. It can be tempting and common for a variety of reasons to just try to pretend that your argument is fine even when you know that it isn't. You may feel discouraged to think that you have to start all over—this really messes with all of your structured planning. You may also feel like you have come up with a lot of good ideas, and you don't want to lose them.

Nonetheless, we would like to introduce the idea of abandoning your writing in some of these situations. We know that this can be a scary endeavor. However, remember that, at the beginning of this book, we talked about how emotional the process of academic writing can be. All of the work that you have done, even if you don't actually use it, is still helpful because it helped you to realize the argument that you actually need to make. If you do not abandon ship in these instances, you may be trying to force an argument that ultimately just does not work, and your reader(s) will ask you to rewrite it anyway. See Practice Exercise 6.3 to explore when to reorganize, delete, or keep your academic writing.

PRACTICE EXERCISE 6.3. When to Reorganize, Delete, or Keep Your Writing

When you are struggling with a certain direction in your writing, ask yourself the following questions to assess whether you are heading in the correct direction:

Reorganization Questions
- "Would a conversation with a peer or professor help me?"
- "Will a new dive into the literature help me?"
- "Can I use a mind map, Venn diagram, or other brainstorming tool?"

Deletion Questions
- "Where are the leaps in my writing?"
- "Where does my writing lack specificity?"
- "Am I holding on to parts of my writing because I do not want to start over?"

Keep Questions
- "Does my writing support my overall argument?"
- "Is there a logical flow of my writing from sentence to sentence, paragraph to paragraph, and section to section?"
- "Do I have adequate evidence to support the conclusions in my writing?"

As we mentioned earlier, for those with a more free-flowing time/space orientation, the messier or less structured parts of the academic writing process will likely be the parts that you find most enjoyable. Your strengths will likely include coming up with ideas, an untiring willingness to look for more and more literature, and an easier ability to change directions if it seems necessary. Your growing edges will most likely be meeting deadlines in a specific sense and maybe something like follow-through in a more general sense. Therefore, for those with a more free-flowing time/space orientation, we recommend the following three strategies for leveraging your free-flowing strengths: Change your attitude toward writing deadlines, use a task-completion approach to writing, and talk through your writing frequently.

1. *Change your attitude toward writing deadlines.* Those of you with a more free-flowing time/space orientation may have a decided dislike for deadlines because they feel like the external impositions of those who are more structured. You may feel that they stifle your flow or creativity. We won't deny that they can definitely feel that way. Of course, focusing on your dislike of deadlines is not going to change the fact that they do exist, and it isn't going to move you forward in your writing process. However, because you are more free flowing, you are likely flexible and find it easier to change, so why not use your strength of flexibility to change your attitude?

Simply accepting that deadlines are an inevitable and unavoidable part of the writing process is an important first step. You are not a bad person or writer if you miss them, nor are you a good person or good writer just because you meet them. However, your relationship with deadlines can affect your relationships with your readers and collaborators, which can ultimately affect your opportunities. So you do need to develop a more positive relationship with deadlines.

We suggest two attitude shifts toward deadlines that might help your free-flowing self find deadlines slightly more palatable. First, try seeing deadlines as "limits" that are there to protect you from yourself. They keep you from working on something too much and too long before seeking feedback. They are put there to keep you from overdoing it, from feeling stressed out about writing all of the time. They are there to allow you to have time to enjoy other parts of your life.

Second, try seeing deadlines as something other people use to protect their personal time and space, so meeting them is like a way of showing courtesy and respect for other people's needs. For example, if you don't meet your deadline and turn something in late, it could interfere with your readers' ability to spend time with their families. Yes, that might lay a guilt trip on you, but it may provide enough of a reasonable rationale for a deadline so that your free-flowing nature can accept the importance of meeting the deadline.

2. *Use a task-completion approach to writing.* Because those with a free-flowing time/space orientation are inherently less focused on measuring time, the idea of trying to schedule specific amounts of time to work on the different aspects of the writing process probably feels very overwhelming. Therefore, we suggest that you look at writing projects as composed of a series of tasks that are in turn composed of a series of steps. Rather than planning based on time, which you probably don't like, try following

a task-completion approach to writing. This approach comprises the following steps:

- Make a list of *all* of the tasks that you need to do in order to finish your written text.

- For each task, make a list of all of the steps that it will take to complete that task. Those steps could be thinking or doing steps. For example, one step might be to "decide" something. Another step might be to "find" something. It's important to keep the steps as small as possible. For example, the task "find articles for lit review" could be divided into four or five smaller steps that all say "find 10 potential articles for lit review."

- Review the small steps that you have listed. Chances are that you can work on smaller steps that are related to different tasks simultaneously.

- Count the days between this moment and your ultimate deadline (actually count the days between now and the day before your deadline to give yourself a small cushion).

- Decide which steps you will do each day between now and then and list those steps according to the day you will do them.

- Beginning with the steps for days 1 and 2 of your list, consider the demands of those days, and write down a general time when you think you can complete that step. Focus only on days 1 and 2 at this point. For example, you could write, "before I go to work" or "while I'm waiting on Nick to finish piano practice." Have a notation system whereby you mark off steps that are fully completed versus those that you worked on but didn't complete. On day 2, spend a few minutes writing down general times for the steps on days 3 and 4. If you're not finishing steps, maybe they aren't small enough. You can break things down into even smaller steps if you need to. However, try very hard to see completing steps as non-negotiable agreements.

- Share your steps for each day with others who share time and space with you and ask them to support and encourage you in accomplishing the steps. If you have a person in your life who is more structured than you but still compassionate about your time/space preferences, you might consider sharing your steps with her and having her help you figure out which steps are realistic for different days.

- Definitely create a writing kit with everything you need for writing that you take with you wherever you go. You may find that you have 30 minutes you didn't expect, and you can possibly complete a step or get started on one if you have everything you need ready to go.

3. *Talk through your writing frequently.* For those who have a more free-flowing time/space orientation, you may be more a talker than a doer

when it comes to writing projects, which may sound like a criticism, but we don't mean it that way. In fact, you can use your willingness to talk about the project to help you move into action. Talking can be a form of doing in which you use your talking to rehearse your academic writing arguments. You can talk your arguments through with anyone who will listen or just talk them through to yourself while you are driving, running, walking, or whatever.

For you, talking will help you to stay consciously immersed in the thinking and writing process of composing your text, which can help you to stay connected to the action aspects of the writing process. This is important because you may have a tendency to disengage with the actions of the writing process easily and then find it hard to reconnect. So, as you are doing anything that allows you the time and space to think about what you want, choose to think about your writing.

Think of the points that you need to make, what the possible counterarguments would be for those points, how you can refute those counterarguments, what evidence you need to support your claims, why any of this matters in your field, and so on. In short, whenever possible, immerse yourself in your writing even when you are not writing. Sometimes even explaining what you are doing to someone who knows nothing about your field can be helpful, because their questions can add a lot of clarity to your explanations. You can even audio-record yourself talking through your topic and listen to this recording later for reminders or inspiration. Talking through your writing and staying connected to your writing process will ultimately pay off by helping you to get started on and finish the steps you have outlined for each day more quickly.

Of course, none of the advice we give can erase the fact that the academic writing process is a time-bound and time-sensitive process. And this will probably create a lot of stress and anxiety for you. You will need to experiment with techniques for managing this in a way that honors your free-flowing nature. There is one more skill that those with more free-flowing time/space orientations may want to develop just to make their academic writing life easier: Know how much time it takes to write.

4. *Know how much time it takes to write.* Being able to estimate about how much time different writing tasks take is extremely helpful and important. From seasoned academic writers to beginners, we have found that most people underestimate the amount of time that it will take them to complete writing tasks. Underestimating the amount of time required to produce academic writing leads to poor-quality writing. For example, we have known plenty of smart students with great ideas, but when they do not set aside the time they need to write well, they set themselves up for disappointment on a couple of levels. First, they receive negative feedback on their writing, which can be discouraging and make them feel as though they do not have good-quality ideas, thus creating self-doubt. This is an

inaccurate assessment when the real issue was inadequate time to produce quality writing. Second, they feel as though they let down their professors or mentors, in addition to themselves. This latter issue can be detrimental to developing positive working relationships with professors and mentors, as turning in poor-quality writing and missing deadlines can create frustration on both sides. With poor-quality writing, your professor and mentors often have to sift through the writing errors, which can obscure an understanding of your good ideas.

So thinking about how much time writing *actually* takes is important. In Box 6.1, you will see a list of what Anneliese has found as average amounts of time that it takes for her to complete various writing activities. Lauren's estimates for how long it takes her would be as much as two times longer.

You may wonder whose times are "correct"—Anneliese's or Lauren's—and the answer is neither. There is no correct amount of time. The important thing is for you to develop a very realistic sense of how long various writing activities take *you*. When you finish a writing project or a task or even just a step, it's important to reflect consciously on how long it really took you to complete it. Make a note of that amount of time, and the next time you're faced with the same project, task, or step, use those real data as part of your plan. Although optimistic or wishful thinking can make you feel temporarily better in the writing process, ultimately a writing plan built on a realistic sense of how long things take you will make you feel best because it will allow you to finish on time. Use Practice Exercise 6.4 to begin figuring out how long it takes you to complete different writing tasks.

BOX 6.1. Average Completion Times for Anneliese

- Reading a 20-page article: 30–40 minutes.
- Writing an abstract: 30–40 minutes.
- Creating a table of information: 20–40 minutes.
- Writing a 10-article (20 pages each) annotated bibliography: 2–3 hours.
- Writing one double-spaced page of academic writing: 20–60 minutes.
- Writing a three-page literature review: 2–3 hours.
- Responding to one single-spaced page of professor feedback: 3–5 hours.
- Proofreading and correcting my writing for grammatical and style errors, typos, awkwardly written sentences, lack of clarity and cohesion, etc.: 1–2 hours.

PRACTICE EXERCISE 6.4. How Long Does It Take You?

1. Think about a writing project that you recently finished.
2. Make a list of the tasks (divided into smaller steps) that you had to complete to finish the project.
3. For each step, list the real amount of time that it took to complete the step.
4. Add up the total time for each task and the total time for the entire project.
5. What time challenges did you encounter while completing this task?
6. Considering the real times that you spent on the steps, what advice would you give to your future self if you were faced with a similar writing project? (Be specific in your advice—don't just say, "Start sooner.")

Personal Coping Style

With regard to academic writing, we think of your personal coping style as the deeply embedded personal preferences you have toward risk taking and feedback. We see risk taking and feedback as two parts of a single process, and, like time, they are unavoidable and inevitable aspects of the academic writing process. All academic writers must take the risk of writing down their ideas and sharing those ideas with known and unknown readers. And, as we have discussed, those readers are understood to be critical readers in the sense that they are looking for flaws or weaknesses in the writer's argument. It is part of the reader's job (in many cases) to provide a critique of the written text in the form of feedback, which can feel a lot like criticism.

As we see it, there is a continuum of personal coping styles for the risk-taking–feedback process of academic writing that might have "plays it safe" at one end and "lets it all hang out" at the other end. Of course, writers may find themselves at any point along this continuum, and where they fall may vary according to the writing project and the reader.

If you are more in the direction of a play-it-safe writer, you are probably a person who likes to avoid risks by knowing exactly what is expected of you. You probably read directions carefully and schedule appointments with your professors just to clarify your understandings of what you are supposed to do. You also probably seek confirmation from your professors that you are on the right track as you move through the writing process. For example, you may be a person who wants to discuss your writing plans and ideas with your professor quite often. Your motivation for avoiding risks is likely related to your desire to avoid negative or what you may perceive as negative feedback.

If you are more in the direction of a lets-it-all-hang-out writer, you probably like the challenge a risk poses. You may like to figure things out as you go, and you're not overly preoccupied with understanding or meeting expectations. You likely are not that concerned with making mistakes because you figure that the professor will let you know what you need to fix. You are probably open to feedback and see it as part of a natural learning process that involves trial and error.

Both coping styles have their strengths and growing edges with respect to academic writing. The person who plays it safe is likely very careful and intentional in the planning and writing of his texts. In addition to checking in with his professors frequently before and during the writing, this person is probably highly attentive to any models that have been provided and is careful to follow those models. The person who plays it safe is likely to follow any and all writing guidelines to the letter. However, a person with this coping style can become overly concerned with "doing it right" and/or pleasing a specific reader in his effort to avoid negative feedback. This can be an obstacle to the actual process of getting started (i.e., writing that first draft), and it can also result in writing that lacks a strong sense of voice.

The lets-it-all-hang-out writer may be an excellent ideas person. Big-picture brainstorming is likely something that comes easily to this type of writer. The lets-it-all-hang-out person probably does not concern herself with checking in with her professors to see if she has it "right." Rather, she enjoys the creative freedom of working autonomously and may take creative liberties in her interpretations of any models and guidelines that may have been provided. However, the written texts of people with this coping style may come across as unfinished (e.g., poorly written due to lack of editing and/or not well thought out due to gaps in the argument), because the lets-it-all-hang out writer is "counting on" the reader's feedback to help her finish the text. The lets-it-all-hang out writer may appear irresponsible or unconscientious to readers because she does not appear to be turning in the best work possible. These writers may overly burden readers by relying on them so much to "fix" their writing through the feedback they provide.

Even though we have described the personal coping styles for the risk-taking–feedback process of academic writing as a continuum, which may imply that you are mostly one or the other, we have observed that there are many student writers who appear to be right in the middle of that coping-styles continuum. They do play it safe in the sense that they are feedback-averse. They pay attention to guidelines and models in an effort to do it "right," but they may be overly focused on the superficial aspects of those guidelines and models; you might describe them as focusing more on the letter of the law than the intent of the law. However, they also let it all hang out in the sense that they may go their own way without clarifying their understandings or discussing their writing plans with their professors. This can result in writing that does not properly anticipate and answer the reader's objections. Instead, the writing may appear to go off on somewhat off-topic tangents that are reflective of a more self-focused than other-focused approach to writing.

The primary strength of the play-it-safe coping style is that the writer is aware of the written text as an understanding that is created collaboratively between the writer and the reader, and these writers are attentive to *how* this collaboration is created. The primary strength of the lets-it-all-hang-out coping style is that writers are not afraid to share their ideas with readers, and they *willingly* accept that feedback and revision based on that feedback are part of the writing process. Oddly, the strengths of both coping styles lead us to suggest the same strategy for leveraging your strengths: Use peer writing groups. However, even though we suggest the same strategy for both coping styles, we do think that the strengths and growing edges of each coping style will benefit from different types of peer writing groups. For the plays-it-safe writer, we suggest using face-to-face peer writing groups, and for the lets-it-all-hang-out writer, we suggest online peer writing groups.

1. *Use face-to-face peer writing groups.* For the play-it-safe coping style, participating in a face-to-face peer writing group is a great way to get nonthreatening feedback that helps you to clarify your understandings and address your concerns about being on the right track. Peer writing groups that you can join may already exist within your department, university, or community, or you may want to start a writing group of your own. Importantly, peer writing groups do not have to necessarily be peers that are in your discipline. In fact, sharing your writing with peers who generally understand your field but are not necessarily in your discipline can result in feedback that really strengthens your argument, because they may see gaps that you are overlooking because you are assuming too much about the reader. As long as the peers are academic writers in similar enough fields, they know or are learning what readers want to see and not see in arguments, so their technical knowledge of your discipline may not be all that necessary for providing valuable writing feedback.

As we mentioned, writers with a play-it-safe coping style are typically very concerned with "getting it right" in terms of how they build collaboration with the reader, and they would also like to avoid negative feedback from their evaluative readers (e.g., professors). Having a group of supportive intermediary readers such as a face-to-face peer writing group can help with both of these concerns.

These types of peer writing groups come in all shapes and sizes, and they work most effectively when they fit how you work best. If you are the kind of writer who really does not want to risk too much in terms of time and effort without knowing that you are going in the right direction, forming a peer writing group of people who actually get together to write might work best for you. For example, you might join or form a small peer writing group that has regular meeting days and times in a specific place where your members get together and write separately on different projects. These meetings might begin with a brief check-in during which members briefly describe the projects they are working on and the parts of the projects they are currently writing. The group can agree to write for a specific amount of time, say 2 hours. After 2 hours, the members can check back in and share their work for immediate feedback. In this way, your risk is minimal, and you get a sense of how you are doing before you have gone too far.

If face-to-face peer writing groups that include writing and feedback in situ don't appeal to you or seem impractical, you can, of course, form or join a peer writing group in which people share their writing in the group (or possibly before the group meets) so that the time spent in the group is strictly for the discussion of feedback. To improve everyone's sense of "safety" in the group, you might consider having a group protocol for providing feedback, such as that everyone begins and ends their feedback with something they liked about each peer's text and/or something they felt that their peer was doing well in their text. For the play-it-safe coping style, hearing about what is being done "right" or well is just as important as hearing about what needs to be improved. See Box 6.2 for a description of Anneliese's peer writing group experience.

BOX 6.2. "I Love My Peer Writing Group."

I have been in a writing group for nearly a decade with two peers who are in very different disciplines (early childhood education, recreation and leisure studies) from me (counseling). Our group elected to meet every 6 weeks, give or take, and to share our writing with one another the week before the writing group meets. Then, in the writing group, we all share the feedback we have on one another's writing. At the end of the writing group, we conclude by setting our next writing goal. During the time of the writing group, we have published numerous articles, chapters, books, letters to the editor, opinion pieces, and more. Our university even wrote an article about some of our success – here is an excerpt:

> The three soon realized they shared a similar interest in feminist research methods. Once back on campus, they formed a writing group to provide each other critical feedback on manuscripts, grant submissions and, later, promotion and tenure materials. . . . "We have held one another accountable for rigorous writing and submission goals," Jones said. "This has resulted in very high levels of production and quality in our scholarship including many books, top-tier journal articles, editorships, keynote presentations and awards. We all believe that our writing group has been the key to our successful writing trajectories, as we have become trusted colleagues and friends who support one another well beyond the sphere of writing." (University of Georgia Office of Vice President for Public Service and Outreach, 2014).

Pretty cool, eh? Academic writing can even help you make some of the best friends you will ever have in your life.

—Anneliese

2. *Use online peer writing groups.* For writers with the lets-it-all-hang-out coping style, we recommend online peer writing groups rather than face-to-face groups for a couple of reasons. First, the lets-it-all-hang-out writers may do lots of creative composing in their heads that they never actually put into written words, which means that they may prefer talking about what they are going to write more than actually writing it. If these writers are in a face-to-face peer writing group, they may get caught up in theoretical discussions of what they will write versus practical discussions of what they have written.

Second, the lets-it-all-hang-out writers are typically not feedback-averse, as they tend to view trial and error as part of the process and kind of expect readers to provide feedback that will improve their writing. As anyone who has ever read the online comments posted in response to such things as articles and blogs will tell you, what people say online and what they would likely say in person are remarkably different. For better or for worse, the keyboard seems to enhance people's directness. Peer responses to written texts online will undoubtedly be more pointed and direct than they would be in a face-to-face situation. If you have a lets-it-all-hang-out coping style, this is actually a good thing, because your future evaluative readers (e.g., professors) would actually like for you to tighten things up a bit before you give them your work. This kind of feedback is probably exactly what you need, and it is better for you to receive this feedback and address it *before* you give your text to evaluative readers. Initially, you may doubt your peers' feedback and think they are off-base, but over time, we predict that you will come to see that if you don't follow your peers' feedback on these matters, your evaluative reader will give you the same feedback.

One of the benefits of an online group is that you can create or join a group of peers who may be anywhere. Another is that there's no need for everyone to show up at the same time in the same place. Everyone can compose their writing and provide feedback on others' writing in their own preferred spaces according to their own schedule. Of course, an online peer writing group only works if you do have some agreements about when submissions will be made and when feedback will be delivered. In order to maintain an online group, honoring commitments like those is super-important, because people may find it easier to exit an online peer group than a face-to-face one if they feel that they are not getting a return on their investment. For example, a peer group of four may agree that a specific person submits work a certain week by Monday and that this work is returned with feedback by the other three peers by Friday. Then, the next Monday, a different person submits his work, and so on. Given the fact that the writer with a let-it-all-hang-out coping style may be less attentive to details than perhaps he should be, it would be best to form an online group with peers who are willing to point this out rather than a group who might be trying to spare each other's feelings.

The challenging thing might be figuring out how to find or set up an online peer group. Social media could be a great way to advertise that you are looking for an online peer writing group. If you put it out there, chances are that someone you know may know someone who may be interested in joining the group or may know someone who is. You may also be able to reach out to peers whom you have met at conferences, in previous degree programs, or even in online courses you may have already taken. You don't need a huge group of people. In fact, three to four people in a group should do it, provided that everyone honors their commitments.

As a bonus, you may find that the accountability check of knowing that there are people waiting to see your work may inspire you to move more quickly from the strictly mental composing process to the actual physical composing process (i.e., fingers on the keyboard). And, as another bonus, providing peer feedback will likely improve your own writing because you learn to see your own writing more critically as you provide feedback on others' writing. It can lead to internal "aha!" moments; you may be engrossed in some sort of commentary, such as "I cannot believe this person did this or did not do that," and then you think, "Oh, wait a minute, I think I do that. Maybe that isn't a good idea when I do it, either."

Just as we have proposed that the strengths of the plays-it-safe and lets-it-all-hang-out coping styles lend themselves to the use of the same strengths-based strategy—peer writing groups—albeit in different forms, we also think that the growing edges of each coping style suggest that both coping styles might consider developing similar long-term skills, again for different reasons, to make their academic writing experiences easier over the long haul. These skills include the following: Just get it out and manage your response to feedback.

1. *Just get it out.* Both the plays-it-safe and the lets-it-all-hang-out coping styles may wind up coping with their respective overfocus and underfocus on "getting it right" by not doing anything. That is, writers with either style may find that simply beginning to physically write is a gigantic obstacle. One group may not be able to begin because they are overly concerned with the evaluative reader (e.g. the professor), and the other group may not be able to begin because they are so unconcerned about their responsibility to the reader. (They could also simply be unaware.) In either case, just getting it out—and by *it* we mean the first draft—could be really hard.

For the plays-it-safe coping style, we think following Anne Lamott's (1995) advice is useful. Lamott talked about the ways that our inner writing critic gets us discouraged from writing at all. This inner critic is the voice that tells us we can't write, so why should we even start? She asserted that in order to tame this inner critic, the strategy of writing "shitty first drafts" can help. Besides being a little hilarious, we have found that when student writers, especially those with the plays-it-safe coping style, use this approach, they are able to rein in that inner critic's voice.

Writing a "shitty first draft" really refers to the idea that if you are pressuring yourself to write perfectly the first time you write, you may be discouraging yourself. Writing a poor first draft means that, every time you tell yourself something doesn't make sense or isn't good, you acknowledge that inner critic and keep on writing anyway—thereby producing more writing. The most surprising thing those play-it-safe student writers find when they give themselves permission to write a terrible first draft is that their writing isn't terrible at all. So the skill to develop if you are of the play-it-safe ilk is the ability to coach yourself mentally to just get it out even if you think it's no good. Don't stop writing. You can always revise later, and remember the entire point is to get your writing down on the page and move you forward to getting your writing done.

If you have a lets-it-all-hang-out coping style, you may also have a hard time just getting it out, but we don't recommend the "shitty first draft" for you. You will likely also struggle with getting started, and what you turn in may not actually be that good because you underestimated what was expected of you as the writer and overestimated the role that your evaluative readers wanted to play in improving your writing (i.e., you thought that they wanted to help you rewrite your first draft). To be clear, your evaluative readers (e.g., professors, editors, collaborators) do not really want to see your first attempt at something. They expect that they will need to provide feedback to improve what you have submitted, but they don't expect that they will need to rewrite your text or remind you of things that may have already been spelled out in guidelines or instructions that you received. So this means that you actually need to do several drafts *before* you submit it to your evaluative reader rather than submitting the first one you actually transcribed from your brain to the keyboard.

For the let-it-all-hang-out coping style, the idea of multiple drafts may seem unnecessary, but we assure you that your evaluative readers really do not want to see your first draft as your supposed best work for them to evaluate. For you, the just-get-it-out skill you need to develop is some type of accountability mechanism that will motivate you to get the first draft out ahead of time so that you can actually work on improving your writing before you submit it for evaluation. The exact accountability mechanism you use for just getting it out depends on your personality and what works for you. Some people use social media such as Facebook. They post a writing goal for their friends to see and ask their friends to check in with them about it. The semipublic nature of this type of accountability mechanism can be highly motivational to some. Of course, you could achieve the same thing privately by setting writing goals with a friend and having the friend text you at a specific time to see what you have done. Whatever mechanism you use, we simply suggest that for the let-it-all-hang-out coping style, it is important to just get a first draft out *before* your first draft is your final draft, so find a mechanism that works for you.

2. *Manage your response to feedback.* As we mentioned earlier, writing involves risk taking. You must risk sharing your writing, knowing that the evaluative reader is going to provide at least some critical feedback. The

coping styles that we have been discussing have different relationships to critical feedback. The writer with the plays-it-safe style basically tries to do everything she can to avoid it, and the writer with the lets-it-all-hang-out style basically accepts that it is inevitable and doesn't do as much as she could to avoid it. Emotionally, feedback can be hard on both coping styles. For example, it may be painful to one group and overwhelming to the other. For both coping styles, we suggest that learning how to manage feedback is a skill that could not only improve their writing but also their confidence.

Receiving feedback from professors, peers, colleagues, journal reviewers, and more is one of the most challenging aspects of writing. This can be inherently frustrating for two major reasons. First, the developmental stage of your academic writing sets the stage for the type of feedback you receive. Whether you are a beginning, intermediate, or advanced academic writer reflects a different understanding of your own academic voice. For beginning academic writers, more support is needed in mastering the basics of academic writing. For instance, with newer academic writers, we consistently provide feedback on the following:

- Articulating a rationale.
- Strengthening literature review.
- Use of manuscript style guidelines (e.g., APA style, Chicago style).
- Replacing speaking language terms with more formal academic writing terms.

With academic writers at an intermediate stage, the feedback we provide tends to move beyond the basics of use of style and writing literature reviews:

- Weaving the rationale throughout the entire manuscript.
- Integrating recent literature.
- Synthesizing literature.
- Critiquing literature.

For advanced academic writers who have proficiency in the above, we typically provide feedback that deepens the use of personality within their academic voices:

- Exploring rationale building in relation to one's overall research agenda.
- Critique literature while drawing in support from one's own research.
- Decreasing sentences with citations.
- Increasing the use of the writer's own thinking.

No matter which level of academic writing you find yourself at, each level reflects the building blocks needed to develop your own writing voice.

The second consideration when receiving feedback from others entails understanding *who* is providing the feedback and *what* the expectations are for integration of the feedback offered. For instance, professors will likely give feedback to students that should be integrated—unless there is a misunderstanding in the professor's reading of your argument or topic. You are typically better off integrating this feedback, as the professor is most likely expecting you to do so, since he took the time to provide the feedback to you. Peers and colleagues, on the other hand, may provide feedback that they may not expect you to integrate into your writing. It is the same with journal reviewers: There may be feedback offered, but it is up to you whether you address the feedback or not.

In most cases, however, we would like to offer some rules for the road on what to do with feedback on your academic writing. Ask yourself the following questions to assess your next steps:

- Who is giving you the feedback?
- Are you expected to integrate the feedback?
- How will integrating the feedback influence or shift your overall argument and/or topic?
- Do you agree with the feedback? Why?
- Are there portions you do not agree with due to your overall argument and/or topic? Why?
- How long will it take you to address the feedback in your manuscript?

We call these rules for the road because we don't think you can go wrong by asking yourself these questions in any situation in which feedback is given on your academic writing. We also think it is helpful to keep a running list separately of the feedback you have addressed, as well as the feedback you have not addressed. Below is an example from a reviewer of one of our journal articles. Notice that we listed the reviewer's comments first, and then placed our response to the comments in italics:

Comment 1: The literature on the construct of resilience should cite the original source.

- *We cited Masten (2001) as the original source of our definition of resilience.*

Comment 2: I would suggest the research question be listed in the Method section, not at the end of the literature review.

- *We made this change.*

Comment 3: Why is literature on discrimination added? This seems off-topic for your study on resilience.

- *Our study of resilience specifically examined the resilience participants had in response to discrimination experiences.*

> *Therefore we believe the literature reviewed on discrimination is necessary to set the rationale for our study.*

You can see that there were comments the reviewer made that we believed would strengthen our study in terms of the overall argument and topic, and we said that we made a change. However, you also should note that when we disagreed with the feedback, we provided a clear reason related to our topic and rationale of why we were not going to make the change. This type of approach—listing the comments and providing your responses—builds a relationship with the people providing feedback on your academic writing. Certainly, not all situations in which you receive feedback will require this formality, including feedback from peers and colleagues. However, we do believe in working with professors, and this can be a helpful road map for them. They likely have been providing lots of feedback to many different people. Your listing of your comments and your responses can not only remind them of where you are in your manuscript development but also serve as an accountability measure to assess where you are and where you are going.

This brings us to the emotional part of receiving feedback. Yes, we have said repeatedly that writing is an emotional venture. So we want you to feel prepared to receive feedback and not shrink from it, put off reading it, or get overwhelmed. This is why it is important to use the questions we have given you above to assess any writing feedback. We also recommend that you open and read feedback *as soon as possible* when you receive it. We have watched as many students and academic writers have postposed reading a review of their work, anxious about the enormity of the feedback, when only about an hour's worth of work was required.

Of course, we cannot promise you that all feedback will only take an hour for you to respond to. However, we can promise you that when you read the feedback right away and take a few notes to develop a plan of response, you will feel more prepared and less stressed because you just closed an "open loop." What is an open loop, you ask? Research on productivity and stress management has asserted that each time we are given a task to do, this creates an open loop of mental energy that has nowhere else to go (Allen, 2002). You can think of this as that "hanging-over-your-head" feeling that academic writing projects often seem to engender! The good news is that this research has also asserted that if you do something to close the loop, the brain can rest. To close the loop on integrating feedback, do the following as soon as possible:

- Schedule a short time on your calendar to review the feedback.
- Schedule a longer time on your calendar than you think you will need to attend to the feedback.

Then, once you are in that longer scheduled writing session attending to feedback you have received, if you find yourself needing more time to work, go on and schedule your next writing block. In each of these steps, you have closed the loop, letting your brain feel assured that there is time on the calendar when you will work. You get the idea. The biggest challenge, of course, is treating your scheduled writing time like a doctor's appointment. (Actually, it might feel that way—not your favorite activity!) Treat your writing calendar as sacredly as you would your health appointments. Show up, and then write. Each time you do this, you develop trust in yourself that you can keep your promises to yourself. You also further develop your writing voice and skills each time you show up at these writing appointments. And, as we have said with academic writing, the little steps matter—and become giant leaps in your overall confidence and mastery of academic writing.

Personal Motivation

In terms of writing, we think of personal motivation very simply as your current feelings about the writing task at hand. As you might have guessed, we would say there is a continuum between the extremes of "I want to do this" and "I don't want to do this," and clearly you are not always at the same point, as many factors can influence your motivation. In the case of personal motivation, we look at being closer to the end of the I-want-to-do-this feeling as a strength and being closer to the end of the I-don't-want-to-do-this feeling as a growing edge. Obviously, being closer to the I-want-to-do-this end of the continuum offers you the great advantages of increased willingness, focus, energy, commitment, and persistence, which are all highly desirable for writing. On the other hand, being closer to the I-don't-want-to-do-this end depletes you of these same qualities, which clearly creates obstacles for writing.

Although many of the strategies and skills we have already discussed in this chapter could be useful for shifting you closer to the strengths-based end of the continuum (i.e., "I want to do this"), we also think the following two strategies can be useful: Develop the ability to *honestly* assess your own motivation and find ways to integrate creativity into your academic writing process.

1. *Develop the ability to honestly assess your own motivation.* Most people think motivation is something that you should just be able to drum up if you need it. However, that isn't exactly how it works. Just having goals and a positive attitude about your task, which many think is motivation, may not be enough (in fact, some research says these things are actually insufficient to bolster motivation). Motivation is something more—it includes practices that you cultivate over time. Motivation also includes how much you believe in your ability to do something. In formal terms, this is called your *self-efficacy*. So take a moment to answer the following question, and scale your answer on a 0–10 scale, with 1 being "not so much" and 10 being a hearty "yes." We will call this your self-efficacy writing scale:

How much do you believe in your ability to do academic writing?

Self-efficacy influences our motivation for sure. So, if you are in the 3 and below range, your motivation is going to be on the low side with academic writing; a range of 4–6 puts you squarely in the middle of motivation to complete a task; and 7–10 has you on the up side of feeling motivated to bring a task to completion.

Motivation is also related to the willingness to do the work of academic writing, so we like to ask students to scale themselves from 0–10 on the following question as well when assessing motivation:

> How willing are you to learn how to become a better writer and put the skills you learn into practice?

So, right now, scale yourself in response to this question, with below 3 on the low side of willingness to learn and implement skills, 4–6 right in the middle of this learning and implementation, and 7–10 meaning you have higher levels of willingness to learn and improve your academic writing.

Once you have asked yourself both of these questions, you end up with what we like to call your current motivation in regard to academic writing. It is an easy-to-use formula to assess your motivation. The formula goes like this:

$$\text{Self-efficacy} \times \text{Willingness to practice} = \text{Current motivation}$$

For instance, let us say you arrive at your planned writing time with an 8 on the second question of willingness to learn and improve your academic writing skills, but you are not feeling particularly strong in your ability to do academic writing that day and you rate yourself a 0 in this area. In this scenario, you end up with a 0 in terms of your current motivation, because the lack of self-efficacy to do academic writing cancels out your willingness to improve your academic writing skills. On that particular day, are you likely to write? Nope. And that may be okay. You may actually need a break. But before you take that break from your writing, ask yourself how you can move up on the self-efficacy scale, because that is how you are going to up your chances for actually putting words on a page that day. Maybe you need to put in a call to your support team—a writing group, your professor, a peer, or your friends and family to remind you that you can write. Maybe you can look back at some previous positive feedback you have received to increase your self-efficacy. Maybe you can shift what you had planned to do that day (e.g., write three pages) to something that you have higher self-efficacy about (e.g., find six articles) instead. This is how you increase your motivation to actually write that day. Do not try to move from a 0 to a 10. Make small moves, from a 0 to a 1 and so forth, so you are realistic and do not overwhelm yourself and end up not writing at all.

So let us talk about another scenario. Let's say your self-efficacy is high (7), but your willingness to learn and improve your writing is low (3).

This often happens when you receive feedback that feels confusing or out of your current wheelhouse. You may begin thinking, "Oh, I'm just lazy today. I'll write later." However, we encourage you to think again of what action you can take to move up that scale of being willing to learn and improve your writing in that moment before you decide not to write. For instance, if you have received feedback that is too general or unclear from your professor, make a list of the changes you can make during that writing session, email your questions to your professor, or make an appointment to see your professor the following week so you can get some clarity. If you have so much feedback that you are wondering how you can get it down, make a list of the changes and go for tiny changes first (e.g., finding typos and grammatical errors, attending to style issues, updating references) so you can build some momentum. Scale yourself again once you are done so you can see where you are now. See Practice Exercise 6.5 to scale yourself right now for one of your current writing projects.

PRACTICE EXERCISE 6.5. Identifying Your Motivation for Academic Writing

Think of a writing project you have on your plate right now. Answer the following questions to scale yourself from 0 (low) to 10 (high):

- How willing are you to learn how to become a better writer and put the skills you learn into practice?
- How much do you believe in your ability to do academic writing?

Plug these two numbers into the equation below to identify your current motivation:

Self-efficacy × Willingness to practice = Current motivation

Identify two to three strategies you could use to move your numbers up on both the self-efficacy and willingness to practice scales.

2. *Find ways to integrate creativity into your academic writing process.* In addition to factors such as self-efficacy and willingness, your motivation to write can be strongly affected by how interesting or uninteresting you find the task or topic at hand. Academic writing can be tedious, boring, and isolating, to name but a few descriptors that might come to mind in your less motivated moments. We think that finding ways to integrate some creativity into your writing can breathe some life into those less motivated moments. (You may need to do a little reframing of your definition of creativity to make this work.)

For example, as we stated early on, academic writing is its own language, so you are likely coming across new words, expressions, and ways of saying things all of the time. Finding ways to work these new language constructs into your own writing can be a motivating creative endeavor (we told you that this might require a reframing of your definition of creativity). It poses a challenge, requires some skillful and strategic decision making, and leaves you feeling very satisfied with yourself. It may sound kind of silly, but actually this kind of "wordplay" really does keep things interesting. So keep a list of words or expressions that you've never used that you would like to try. When your motivation feels depleted while you're writing, massage it by trying to find a way to use one or more of these words or expressions in your writing.

Like wordplay, forced decision making is another reframing of creativity that may help you when your motivation is running low. In some cases, having limited choices results in a more creative outcome. You have to think and plan more carefully and creatively when you have limited choices precisely because you have limitations. You can use the idea that having limited choices leads to greater creativity when you feel stuck in your writing by obligating yourself to do some forced decision making. For instance, if you feel stuck over what are the most important points in an article you want to integrate into your literature review, force yourself to use the "rule of threes" and select the three most salient points. Just say to yourself, "If I could only use three points from this article in my review, what three points should those be and why?" The process of figuring that out will get your creative juices flowing because your brain will be busy creating possible connections between that article and your review to assess which three ideas you should choose. This will shift your focus from the multiplicity of points in the article to the actual support that your writing needs.

You can identify other examples of creativity in your discipline as you read articles, looking for how authors might use creativity in the titles of their papers or in how they structure their overall writing. For instance, Anneliese likes to use participants' quotes in the titles of her research articles. She also has mad love for any opportunity to create a Top-10 list summarizing recommendations or implications in her writing.

Integrating creativity in your writing might also mean switching types of writing. If you have been focusing on a research tradition, such as grounded theory, throughout most of your research and literature reviews, then delving into first-person autoethnographies of research can break up the monotony of consuming one type of research. You can also try reading in a different discipline on a related topic to identify what is going on outside of your field. Breaking up the monotony like this can also help you identify new patterns within or across your discipline.

Creativity can also be increased just by paying attention to your writing environment. Posting quotes and excerpts about writing or about your writing topic by people you admire can be motivating to look at as you write.

You may be someone who likes to have a very soothing environment when you write, and we have known many students who have a designated favorite writing candle that they light only when they write. Others like a more dynamic writing environment, with music in the background or in a public setting where there is a lot to see. Know what you tend to like so you can invite that creativity into your writing process and, in so doing, shift yourself toward the "I want to do this" end of the personal motivation continuum.

Voices in Your Head

As a personal consideration that affects writing, *voices in your head* refers to your past experiences with writing, specifically academic writing. As we all know, past experiences have a significant impact on things like our self-efficacy. When we are metaphorically hearing applause, we tend to perform better, try harder, and take more risks. When we are hearing gremlins (i.e., imaginary, mischievous sprites that cause problems), everything is more difficult. We doubt ourselves and are less open and sometimes even less able to learn.

Although you cannot change your past experiences, you can exert some influence over those voices in your head. As with motivation, you can shift yourself more toward the strengths-based position of hearing applause versus hearing gremlins. We recommend developing the following two skills or habits to accomplish this shift: Take on the gremlins impeding your writing and celebrate your growth as a writer-researcher.

1. *Take on the gremlins impeding your writing.* So let's say you have committed to being your own writing coach, setting solid goals, and rewarding yourself for meeting them. Awesome. In the process, though, there are often little "gremlins" that arise that impede your writing. Gremlins are different from the everyday challenges that can arise in meeting your writing goals, such as family responsibilities or work obligations. We use the idea of gremlins to refer to the deeper core thoughts and beliefs that tend to be negative and lead you down the road toward throwing in the towel on your academic writing. The core thoughts and beliefs lead to frustration and feeling stuck. These gremlins reflect the most negative parts of our thinking about writing and our ability to write. Gremlins also represent the ultimate escape from academic writing. Their only goal is to get in the way of your writing and stop the writing process. Therefore, we want you to be able to identify what your typical writing gremlins are and when they typically arise.

Here are a few pretty typical gremlins that can come up in the writing process. Note which ones sounds familiar to you:

- "I don't know how to write."
- "I should have started writing earlier."
- "I don't really know what I am trying to say."

- "I don't know what to write next."
- "I am never going to finish."
- "Everyone else is a better writer than me."
- "I am a terrible writer."
- "I never learned how to write."
- "If I don't write well, I will fail."
- "I don't know if I am accurately representing my ideas."
- "I don't have enough citations and references."
- "What if I am not putting things in my own words enough?"
- "What if I can't think of any more ideas?"
- "How am I ever going to get this done?"
- "I don't have anything important to say anyway."
- "Who am I to say anything?"
- "Nobody is ever going to read this anyway."
- "I wonder what is going on with my Facebook friends."
- "I hate this [what I am writing]."

And this is just a partial list of common gremlins. You may have specific gremlins related to your writing experience. For instance, you may have been told you were not a good writer when you were in fifth grade, and the gremlin thought of "I can't really write" comes with a gremlin face of your fifth-grade teacher that is tough to shake out of your head.

The thing about gremlins, though, is that we all have them, and they all have the purpose of derailing our progress and making our writing process less enjoyable. So the key is not only to identify them but also to then have strategies for quickly clearing the gremlins out of our writing way. How do you do the clearing? We shorten the time between when we can identify that a gremlin is present and threatening our writing process and the time at which we disinvite it from our heads. Here are the formulaic steps:

- Identify that a gremlin is present (e.g., "My writing is making no sense!").
- As soon as you can, ask yourself, "Do I really want to believe my writing is making no sense?" (Hint: the answer should be no.)
- As soon as you can, ask yourself, "Do I really want this gremlin to hang around as I try to write?" (Hint: the answer should be no.)
- As soon as you can, say to yourself, "Okay—I feel stuck—what do I really need right now?" and do that thing you need for at least 10 minutes (e.g., a break, walk, food, some social time, peer review).
- As soon as you can, tell yourself, "Gremlins are trying to stop me from writing, but they won't win."

- As soon as you can, tell yourself, "I actually have learned a lot about writing and I can get more information if I am truly stuck."
- Commit to making a U-turn toward your writing and away from this annoying gremlin, and identify one next step you can do right now to move ahead (e.g., writing a title page, reading an article, talking to a peer or professor). Sometimes it helps to identify a step that is easy to accomplish (i.e., low-hanging fruit), because finishing that step easily and quickly is likely to begin the process of shutting that gremlin down.

You can see that these formulaic steps start with identifying the gremlins and then focusing on quickly identifying what the real need you have is, taking a short break, and then reminding yourself that you do know a thing or two about academic writing and your topic and that you can get support when you need it in your academic writing. Ultimately, the formulaic steps end with taking a U-turn away from the gremlin and getting back on the writing track, by identifying the very next step that will move you forward.

Although gremlins can feel big, scary, and overwhelming when they appear in the writing process, we have learned to embrace them. We understand now that we are not alone with the gremlins, and the best strategies are the ones that shorten the time until we get to that U-turn away from the gremlins. We have even learned to laugh at our gremlins from time to time. Anneliese knows, for instance, that when the gremlin of "I am never going to finish" arises, she definitely needs to take a walk or listen to some music. Over time, this particular gremlin is almost like an alarm for Anneliese to pause in her writing; the gremlin actually is helpful now because of the related U-turn that she gets to take a break. Lauren knows, on the other hand, that with this same gremlin thought she actually needs to talk through her ideas with a colleague (often Anneliese). In doing so, she uses the gremlin thought to actually keep writing, which is the antithesis of what the gremlin wants. So we challenge you to commit to learning more about what your gremlin thoughts are and how to dodge them as quickly as you can, using them to write even more—and enjoy your writing more. You can explore more in Box 6.3.

BOX 6.3. Gremlin Identification: Getting to the Writing U-Turn

Take out a sheet of paper and divide it into two columns, titled "Gremlin" and "U-turn," respectively. In the left column, list and number all of the negative thoughts and beliefs—the gremlins—that come up for you when you write. In the right column, write a positive, motivating belief or strategy that would work for you when that particular gremlin attempts to get you to stop writing. Talk over your list with a colleague and see if there are additional gremlins and U-turns you need to add to your list.

2. *Celebrate your growth as a writer-researcher.* In addition to banishing gremlins, you can shift the voices in your head in the direction of hearing applause by tracking your growth as an academic writer. There are a few ways you can do this. First, you can think about the first time you ever faced an academic writing project and reflect on how far you have come since that point. Lauren remembers her first academic writing project as a PhD student and how she had no idea what to do. She was changing disciplines and was using writing models from her previous discipline that were not really adding up to success in her new discipline. Since that point she has not only improved in her academic writing year after year, but she wrote her dissertation on teaching academic writing, she currently teaches academic writing to English language learners, and she is writing this book on academic writing. That's a pretty awesome journey, and it is very motivating for her to think about when she gets stuck on a current writing project. She has accomplished so much over time, and tracking her growth helps her stay on track.

Second, you can keep copies of previous writing projects on which you received really helpful or important feedback on your academic writing. Anneliese received some very positive feedback from one of her professors in her doctoral program. She had loved to write creatively—poems and short stories—before her doctoral program. However, making the shift to the formulaic nature of academic writing was a tough transition for her. When she received the positive feedback on her academic writing from her professor, something shifted in her. She realized she could still identify as a "writer," even if she was not doing as much creative writing in her new field. Now, Anneliese is proud to identify as a writer, among her other salient identities, and this identity is a reflection of her growth over time as an academic writer.

A third, and very practical, tracking device is literally to have a journal, notebook, electronic document, or some other place to record your writing accomplishments. This could be a record of feedback you have had on your academic writing—including your strengths and growing edges— across assignments. If you are in a writing group, you could take time to reflect on the number of writings you have all accomplished as a group in 6 months or a year. If you are focused on publishing your writing, then track the numbers and types of publications you have. No matter which of the three strategies you use, when we take time to identify our growth and milestones in our academic writing, we build our confidence for our current and future writing goals and projects. Take a few moments to identify these in Box 6.4.

NAVIGATING REAL-LIFE OBSTACLES TO COMPLETION

Just as there are internal personal considerations that may affect your writing, there are also a host of other external considerations that have

---

BOX 6.4. Identifying Academic Writing Growth and Milestones

For each of the three strategies below, identify how you might integrate the strategy into your life and what strategies might be best at various stages of your career:

1. Self-reflection on your academic writing.
2. Feedback on your academic writing.
3. Track your publishing of academic writing.

---

an impact—including major life changes. You may be in graduate school for several years if you are pursuing a PhD, and your life will change in many ways while you are there. Think about the last 2, 4, or more years of your life and about all the major and minor changes you went through that were expected and unexpected. You are a different person because of these changes, and that is exactly what happens in graduate school. But we find that this is rarely talked about in relation to how this affects getting your academic writing done and completed. In fact, we have actually heard some of our own colleagues advise students not to intentionally make major changes in their lives while they are in graduate school, such as getting married, having children, or traveling abroad.

We think about this a lot differently. We like to think about this issue realistically. Life is too short to wait to make the changes you want or need in your personal life. Plus, you likely already have multiple roles (e.g., partner, child, parent) in addition to your role as a student. So graduate school and academic writing need to fit within your overall life. If you are a caregiver or parent to children or a family member, this is an important part of your life. And then there are the changes you plan to make in your life that are also present. Sure, we acknowledge that if you intentionally plan to make big changes when you are in graduate school, you will necessarily need to think realistically about your timeline for completion. We also believe that if you hold off on some of those big changes that are really important to you, this will ultimately create a kind of battle—graduate school versus your life—that can really sink your progress. The key is to talk through some of these intentional big changes with trusted family, friends, and, of course, your professors and peers. And ask for support when you need it.

On the other hand, there are those big and small changes that happen in your life that are unexpected. Relationships end, people die or get sick, job changes happen, and people move, among others of the top stressors that you can experience in life. In all of these instances, you will necessarily

> ### BOX 6.5. What Staying on Track Really "Looks Like"
>
> As a doctoral student, the first step that I took to ensure I met writing deadlines for classes and my dissertation was to create a writing schedule. For classes and the dissertation, I developed a writing schedule and stuck to it! I found the time of day in which I was most alert—which was early morning for me—and made a commitment to write five days per week for a minimum of two hours. On day six, which was Saturday, I wrote for a longer period of time (approximately 4 hours) and on day seven, I rested and rewarded myself.
>
> Specifically, for the dissertation, I kept the same writing schedule. In addition, I engaged in the writing process (i.e., writing, editing, working on reference page) during every break that I got—whether it was 30 minutes or 15 minutes—I did something. Furthermore, for the dissertation, I created a timeline in which I identified dates that I would complete each dissertation chapter, research, and IRB proposal, and integrated some flex time in the event that something happened to delay my writing time. This timeline was an accountability measure that kept me on track as I progressed towards completing the dissertation. In essence, persevere through tough times, create a schedule and stick to it, celebrate small successes, and engage in the writing process every chance that you get.
>
> —*Lakiesa C. Rawlinson*

need to make shifts in your academic writing. Get the support you need personally, and then make sure some of this support helps you identify when you will return to your writing. Academic writing obviously will not be on the top of your list, and at the same time we want you to have some support on your next steps so that you do not fall into an avoidance trap while you are navigating these larger and more important changes. Regardless of what unexpected obstacle falls in your path, remember that completing academic writing is part of your overall goal of completing your graduate degree. See Box 6.5 to see what staying on track can look like in your life from doctoral student Lakiesa Rawlinson.

CHAPTER SUMMARY AND REMINDERS

In this chapter, we discussed the fact that navigating the academic writing process requires skills beyond just writing. Becoming aware of the personal considerations that may affect the process and understanding how to coach yourself through the process are crucial to your success as an academic writer. In this chapter, we discussed the following specific skills and strategies that we believe may be useful to you in your self-coaching:

- Use a deadline approach to writing.
- Become a regular writer.
- Identify the best places for you to write.
- Be willing to allow your plan to change.
- Change your attitude toward writing deadlines.
- Use a task-completion approach to writing.
- Talk through your writing frequently.
- Know how much time it takes to write.
- Use face-to-face peer writing groups.
- Use online peer writing groups.
- Just get it out.
- Manage your response to feedback.
- Develop the ability to honestly assess your own motivation.
- Find ways to integrate creativity into your academic writing process.
- Take on the gremlins impeding your writing.
- Celebrate your growth as a writer-researcher.

See Summary Table 6.1 for awareness and action reminders.

SUMMARY TABLE 6.1. AWARENESS AND ACTION REMINDERS	
Be aware . . .	Take action . . .
Academic writing is more than a mental process, it is also an emotional process that is affected by a variety of personal considerations.	Be fiercely honest in identifying the personal considerations that affect you.
The best kind of self-coaching for academic writing is positive and strengths-based.	Become a good goal setter.
You can use your strengths to overcome some of your growing edges, and you may need to develop new strengths.	Understand the strengths and growing edges that may affect your writing process and look for strategies that you can use to improve how you navigate the process.

UNIT III
SPECIFIC TYPES
OF ACADEMIC WRITING

Grounding Your Voice in the Literature

A s we have mentioned, successful academic writing is a contradictory mixture of fitting in and standing out within your discipline's CoP. The tension of these contradictions affects the writing process and the process of becoming a writer at multiple points along the way. So you will notice that the chapters in this book may reflect that contradiction as well. For example, it may seem as though we are encouraging you to go your own way in one chapter and sending you back into the pack in another. It is true, because that is actually what we are doing and that is what you have to do as an academic writer. Therefore, you will see in Chapter 7 that the focus is on grounding or situating your voice, particularly the content and approach components of your voice, within the scholarship of your discipline's CoP.

Knowing how to conduct and write up a good literature review is essential in most, if not all, academic disciplines. Our **awareness focus** for this chapter is to help you to develop an understanding of the role that the past (i.e., past research) plays in your success as an academic writer. Our **action focus** includes practical strategies for breaking the tasks of the literature review into manageable parts and putting together a literature review that allows your voice to fit in and stand out.

DEFINING LITERATURE REVIEWS

Situating your voice in relation to the other voices in your field requires you to know the past, which is really what literature reviews entail. You have to know what others have proposed and found in the distant and recent past in relation to the content and approach choices that you have made. In academic-speak, you have to "know the literature." Good academic writing typically requires a strong foundation of literature to support your argument, to counter the ideas of others, to explore a topic, and much more. In fact, any topic or theme that you wish to explore will necessarily begin with a literature review to find out what has already been done.

There are essentially two kinds of literature reviews—the stand-alone literature review and the preamble-to-a-research-study literature review. The stand-alone literature review is a full-length paper or article that reviews lots of literature on a given topic or theme. In Chapter 1, we mentioned that there were four types of research articles: empirical, conceptual, propositional, and responsive. Stand-alone literature reviews are examples of conceptual research. Usually, this kind of stand-alone literature review looks for such things as patterns, gaps, and possible new directions in the literature it reviews. For example, a review of the public health interventions used to respond after Hurricane Katrina in New Orleans would summarize as much literature as possible on any type of public health intervention used to respond to Hurricane Katrina, but it would do something more than summarize, because it would also provide some type of critique or unique point of view in relation to that literature. It would also likely end with a discussion of what is missing in that body of literature and what future directions researchers should consider taking in that area.

A preamble-to-a-research-study literature review is generally shorter. The purpose of this type of literature review is to create a rationale for the research that you are preparing to discuss. It will also review a lot of literature, but it will seek to do so very concisely. Often, this type of literature review includes some discussion of literature that situates your topic in a broader context, as well as discussion of literature that is more specifically related to the study you are doing. For example, if your research focused on measuring the impacts of Hurricane Katrina on the public education system in New Orleans, and your argument was that there were significant negative impacts that had been largely ignored, you would review literature that helped you make this argument. To establish a broader context, that literature might include any research that has been done on the effects of disasters—natural and human-made—on educational outcomes. To establish a more specific context, that literature might include any research that had been done comparing anything education-related (e.g., schools, resources, student achievement) pre- and post-Katrina with a focus on research that showed negative comparisons post-Katrina. You might also review literature that supported the idea that negative impacts of Katrina, whether they related to education or not, had been ignored. The purpose of your review would be to essentially set the stage for the discussion of your research findings.

THE ROLE OF THE LITERATURE REVIEW
IN ACADEMIC WRITING

Think of literature as the history of a topic. Literature essentially represents the historical timeline of development of academic thought on that topic. Huff (1999) likens this timeline or collection of scholarship on a topic to a conversation. Every researcher who wants to establish an academic voice that is attached to that topic needs to learn how to participate in the conversation; in other words, researchers need to become part of the historical *family* of that topic by understanding how the treatment of that particular topic came into being and has progressed over time. It is a sign of respect and humility. After all, you are but one of a long chain of researchers who have addressed or will address this topic in some way. Your credibility in your new family depends upon your appreciating, to some extent, what others have done and continue to do.

Your credibility also depends upon your ability to demonstrate an accurate and thorough understanding of your topic. The only way that other researchers can know whether you accurately and thoroughly understand your topic is by having the opportunity to read your literature review. If your literature review seems reasonable according to their own understandings of the literature you reviewed, your critiques will carry more weight. If, however, your literature review seems flimsy or unfair in its portrayals of other literature, your critiques will be easily dismissed, because it will seem that you do not really have a complete understanding of your topic.

In addition to credibility, literature reviews provide evidence and context for the introduction of your own unique ideas into the historical mix. Literature provides a basis for knowing why your ideas or perspectives are logical next steps in the historical timeline, and this is important. Readers need to be convinced that whatever you are proposing actually represents a growth in the knowledge base of your topic. They need to see evidence from the past organized and explained in a sequence that logically unfolds with your research as the necessary next step. In this way, literature reviews help writers to establish and explain the research gap that they would like to occupy.

Literature reviews also help writers find their voice. Reviewing and explaining past literature helps writers assess their understanding of the research on their topic. As their understanding increases, their ability to offer credible critiques also increases. They begin to form opinions about their topic that are grounded in the literature, and they begin to see what has and has not been studied in relation to their topic. In fact, writing a literature review is a prime example of writing to learn, a concept we mentioned in Chapter 3. Writers literally *learn* what new thing they want to say about their topic by writing about what others have said about it. They find their future by retelling the history of their topic.

So think of writing literature reviews as getting to know your new family while finding your own voice. Think of it as paying your dues to the past while uncovering clues for your own future. Most of all, think of it as the key that opens the door for your voice to be heard.

HUNTING AND GATHERING LITERATURE

The necessary precursor to writing any literature review is the selection of a topic. If you are writing a preamble-to-a-research-study literature review, the topic or topics of the review are dictated by your research questions and, to some extent, your results or findings. If you are writing a stand-alone literature review, topic selection is more complicated, and it can seem overwhelming.

We have seen many student writers struggle with this first step. They choose a topic, begin looking for literature, and find so much or so little that the process overwhelms them. Before your literature search or when feeling overwhelmed by it, having informal conversations with others about the topic of the literature review can be very useful. Conversations with peers allow you to explore what you know and do not know about a topic, and the feedback from your peers may stimulate new and related topics of inquiry or result in good suggestions for ways to find relevant literature. Conversations with professors allow you to get important feedback related to your discipline that can help you narrow your topic selection and focus for your literature review. In addition, professors also frequently know the best search terms to use when looking for literature in databases, and they can direct you to specific researchers who may work in the topic area that you are researching. In Box 7.1, a doctoral student shares her experiences of discussing a literature review with her professor.

Stand-alone literature reviews often begin as wide-angle searches. This means that you may begin by looking for literature on a broad topic. The next time that you are faced with proposing a broad topic for a literature review, have a conversation with a peer or your professor and answer the following questions related to your literature review:

1. "What am I most interested in knowing about in the past scholarship in my discipline?"
2. "What do I think—*just make a guess*—I might find when hunting and gathering literature about this topic?"
3. "What search engines might be helpful to me in identifying past research on this topic?"
4. "What key words might be useful for locating past research on this topic?"

Once you have had these informal conversations with peers and professors and done some wide-angle research, you will have a better idea of

> **BOX 7.1. Words of Wisdom from a Doctoral Student on Selecting a Literature Review Focus**
>
> The most helpful part of the conversations about my literature review with my committee chair involved her knowledge and familiarity with the body of existing literature related to my topic. This allowed us to engage in conversations about the various ideas I had in my head more constructively. Her knowledge of the numerous issues related to my targeted population and the implications associated with researching those issues really helped me see the areas of need as well as ways my research could help improve the life experience of those groups of people. In our conversations, she also asked me what I wanted to do with my research and how I would use what I learned, which allowed me to really assess my goals and therefore make a better decision about my research topic. Make sure to go into your meetings with your professors with an idea of questions you want to ask, and try to complete your "to do" items as soon as you can after your meeting so you can follow up with any clarifying questions and keep writing!
>
> —*Rebecca Eaker*

the directions that the research in your broad topic area takes. You may be able to narrow your topic to something more specific on your own. As you see more and more articles on one topic or a topic that really captivates you, your focus may become clear. However, if the topic is very new to you, you may need to simply bring a few articles that have caught your attention to your professors to see if they can help you narrow your topic.

The search is not over when you narrow your topic. In fact, in many ways, it is just beginning. Now, you need to locate all of the research that you can on your narrowed-down topic. This can be harder, as the key words used to locate that research can be elusive. When looking for literature, you need three important things—time, patience, and determination. Locating and identifying relevant research takes time. Your initial searches—these are the ones you do before you begin writing—will take time, but a literature review also requires ongoing research. You will be looking for and finding research for your literature review before you write it and while you write it. Your hunt for literature will only end when you submit your literature review. However, if you anticipate feedback and rewrites, you will likely continue hunting literature even after submission.

Finding relevant literature also requires patience. There is no magic key term that will produce all of the literature that you need, and there are many places, from books to databases to the Internet, that may lead you to relevant literature. You will also have to contend with the possibilities and limitations of your particular library. You will want and *need* things that it doesn't have. You may be able to get them through procedures such as interlibrary loan, but it takes time.

A thorough search requires determination. You cannot give up after trying only a few search terms. You must persevere, trying different combinations and following different clues that you may be given. You must look at the key search terms that are listed for the articles you have found that seem relevant. You must try those search terms to see where they lead. You must look at the references for articles that seem relevant and go through them to see if any of those references might be important for your literature review. If they are, you must look for them. You must look for things your library does not seem to have in different ways. For example, sometimes your library may not have a book that has a chapter you need in it. If you Google the name of the chapter, you may find that you can gain access to that chapter in some other way.

Once you have settled the question "What is my topic?," you will find yourself at the next question: "Exactly how much literature do I need to review?" If you ask your professor, she may say something not that helpful, such as "Until you have enough articles." This is understandably confusing and discouraging. Your professor is not playing head games with you, we promise. It is just really hard to know how much is enough because enough depends on many factors, such as the type of literature review you are writing, the particular topic that you are researching, and the overall point that you are ultimately planning to make about the literature you review. You definitely have to collect enough literature to actually form and support some kind of meaningful overall point.

Although we kind of agree with your professor's answer to this question, we also think building in some structure to the hunting and gathering of literature can be helpful. So we are going to make a suggestion. Start by setting a goal of finding 10 articles on your narrowed-down topic. Use key words to search for your topic in relevant databases. Look for titles that appear to be related to your topic. Read the abstracts for those articles and consider the relevance that the article has to your topic. And remember that articles are not just relevant because they "agree" with your point of view. It is equally important to find articles that "disagree" with your point of view. At this stage, try to be very strict about deciding relevance; if it is not easy for you to explain the relevance to yourself after reading the abstract, move on to look for other articles. As you search and identify your first 10 articles, you might find that you hit the "mother lode." Hitting the mother lode would mean stumbling upon the exact right combination of key words that provide you with lots of articles on your topic or discovering special issues of journals that are wholly dedicated to your topic. If you hit the mother lode, pull about 10 more articles on your topic.

You could find so many articles right away that you feel overwhelmed with choosing 10. In this case, review your literature focus and concentrate on choosing the ones that are most closely aligned with your literature focus. At the other end of the spectrum, you may start hunting and gathering past research about your topic only to find nothing. Zip. Nada. In these situations, we often see that students have encountered one of two things. First, students may legitimately be in a "gap" in the research. When Anneliese was searching for articles for her dissertation literature review on child sexual abuse and South Asian American women, there was nothing on this particular topic that she found. In these instances, you broaden your scope of research to the next larger related topic. Anneliese then searched for literature related to interpersonal violence and South Asian American women, and, bingo, she hit a mother lode of literature of past conceptual and empirical work in this topic area.

The second reason you may find nothing in the literature is often that your key words for the literature search are too narrow. In these instances, make sure your key words are broad enough to "catch" articles and to search widely enough across disciplines on a certain topic. Using Anneliese's literature review topic example, searching "South Asian American women and child sexual abuse" may bring up a couple of article hits; however, instead of "South Asian American," searching varieties of this term, such as "Indian American" and "South Asian," can be more helpful, just as searching "abuse" or "sexual abuse" might capture more hits than "child sexual abuse." The best news is that, once you find a needed article, it is often easier to find a subsequent article, as many university libraries' computer programs have a search function titled "find similar articles." Your library's program may also have a function that allows you to see who has cited a key article. It is always possible that researchers who are citing an article that is key to your work are writing on topics that are related to your work. See Box 7.2 for some practical words of wisdom from one of Anneliese's favorite librarians, Benn Hall.

BOX 7.2. Words of Wisdom from a Librarian on Keyword Searches in Literature Reviews

The first piece of advice that I give for conducting keyword searches is to break your topic into concepts. A good way to do this is to consider the questions of *who, what,* and *where*? For example, a topic could be broken down into the following three concepts: *high school students,* living with *bipolar disorder,* in *United States public schools.* Next, identify synonyms and related terms for each concept. Then combine these synonyms using the Boolean OR (e.g., guns OR firearms OR weapons). Finally, using an advanced search, combine your concept groups together with the Boolean AND, so that the three concepts will be searched together. Another great tip is to use quotation marks when searching for exact phrases (e.g. "student personnel services").

—Benn Hall

ORGANIZING THE SEARCH

As you gather your articles, you should have a way to manage every piece of information you find. In the quick 10-article-pull strategy we discussed earlier, as you begin to identify these articles, it is helpful to immediately take the time to create electronic folders and subfolders in which you archive these articles. You can begin with creating folders based on your general topics. Then, as you begin to narrow your focus, you can create subfolders of related topics. It is important to rearrange articles as you create new folders. We would also suggest duplicating articles and pasting them in multiple folders if they are related to multiple topics or subtopics. This initial work organizing your literature review search can really pay off later on as you begin later steps in the process.

You should also create some kind of naming conventions for articles that help you to know what they are. It does not help you to have articles named *1234* or *XYZ* or *tdobiyv* or any other nonidentifying names. You need to know the titles and/or topics of your articles at a glance, so take the time to name articles when you archive them.

If you were researching the efficacy of antidepressants and counseling for adults living with depression, you would have two folders you are organizing within your literature review—one on the efficacy of antidepressants with depression and one on the efficacy of counseling with depression. Then, let us say you found several articles that could be shared within these two folders because they were meta-analyses of various studies exploring the efficacy of antidepressants and counseling with depression. These articles could be saved in both folders. You might also have subfolders of these two initial folders that help you distinguish the different types of articles you are finding in your literature review.

If you are crunched for time and are doing a quick literature search for potential topics, but you are not necessarily ready to "commit" to creating subfolders on your computer, you can use the same strategy using a pen and paper. We are fans of having a dedicated notebook, journal, or pad of paper to document ideas, literature searches, conversations, and other activities you may do related to your literature search. As you quickly scan titles and abstracts for relevance to your literature review topic, write down the big areas you are seeing in the literature on this first glance. This strategy can actually be a very helpful one to build confidence in your abilities and get you started on your literature review without much stress. In these instances, your library management system can help you keep track of this initial search, as there are often Web-based folders you can create under your library account. Here are Anneliese's pen-and-paper notes from her initial quick literature review of past conceptual and empirical work on South Asian American women who had experienced child sexual abuse:

1. Used wide variety of keywords as discussed above to identify 10 articles.
2. Identified most of the 10 articles on intimate partner violence that fell into categories of small qualitative studies.
3. Noticed South Asian patriarchal norms, immigration stress, and collectivism were a focus of many articles.
4. Jotted down a note about the three potential categories for future literature searches and for organizing the literature review.

As your literature searches deepen and you identify more and more relevant articles for your topic, you are ready to move into further managing your articles by designing an article tracking system as you read. We like to use an Excel file or Word document to track our literature review articles in a table. This tracking system includes capturing as much information about articles as you can. See Table 7.1, drawn from one of Anneliese's studies on transgender youth and their experiences of school bullying.

In addition to using tables to track your articles in your literature review, we find that when students develop annotated bibliographies, they begin to see deeper connections within the literature base. An annotated bibliography is exactly what it sounds like, as it is a list of brief descriptions of articles. To design an annotated bibliography, you select a number of articles to review. (Why not our magic number of 10?!) Then you list the full reference for the article and follow this with a short description of the article contents.

You can design annotated bibliographies to suit a variety of purposes. You may want to describe your first 10 articles to get your head thinking about your articles a little more deeply, or you may select the more complex articles you have for a deeper read and review. You can also use annotated bibliographies to describe articles that are outside of your discipline or that make a unique contribution to your literature topic. No matter what your purpose is, you can make entries as long or as short as you want.

TABLE 7.1. Tracking Articles for the Literature Review		
Authors	**Article Content or Method**	**Relevance to Topic**
Ahuja et al. (2015)	Conceptual article on LGBTQ youth	Professional organizations serving trans youth discussed links between school bullying and suicide
Wernick, Kulick, & Inglehart (2014)	Quantitative study—multistep linear	Youth-led interventions within peer networks may reduce anti-trans bullying and support trans youth.

We think annotated bibliographies are the most helpful when they do more than just provide a brief summary. Lauren is a fan of annotated bibliographies that include summary + reflection + connection. In this type of bibliography, you briefly summarize the article, state your thoughts or critique of the article, and comment on how this article connects to your topic and/or other articles you have read. When you take the time to create this type of annotated bibliography, you are actually getting ahead in the thinking and writing process because you are "rehearsing" your ideas and your writing. You are practicing the type of summary, synthesis, and explanation that will eventually be included in your literature review. This type of practice always pays off because it helps you to work through the articulation and elaboration process so that later you can write tighter and more concise literature reviews.

When writing annotated bibliographies, make sure to use quotation marks to indicate direct quotes so you know what ideas you have written in your own words and what ideas are direct quotes. Box 7.3 includes examples of annotated bibliography entries for articles related to a literature review on mindfulness. This particular illustration only includes summaries, which might be how the researcher begins the annotated bibliography. As researcher's knowledge of past research increases and his own thoughts about it begin to emerge, the researcher could return to these entries and add reflection and connection commentary.

FOLLOWING THE PRINCIPLE OF RELEVANCE

As we discussed earlier, your review of literature is one of the ways that you establish your credibility in your field. It is one of the ways that others evaluate your true level of knowledge and understanding of your topic. Your decision making is also evaluated. Your decisions to include or not include specific literature in your review demonstrate something about your knowledge and understanding. If the literature you review seems off target (i.e., not related to the point you are trying to make), you will seem less credible. Therefore, it is important to follow the principle of relevance. Following the principle of relevance means being very sure that everything you choose to include or exclude is based on its relative relevance to your topic. It is very easy to lose the principle of relevance during both the research and writing processes, so we think it is important to create an anchor that will hold you steady as you sort through all of the information you are collecting.

As we have mentioned, a literature review begins with the identification of a topic. Then it moves to a narrowing down of the topic to something specific about that topic. At both of those stages, your anchor might be a question. The question would begin as something like "What is known about X?" and change to something like "What is known about x of X?" These questions are anchors in a sea of research information because they

Gayner, B., Esplen, M. J., DeRoche, P., Wong, J., Bishop, S., Kavanagh, L., & Butler, K. (2012). A randomized controlled trial of mindfulness-based stress reduction to manage affective symptoms and improve quality of life in gay men living with HIV. *Journal of Behavioral Medicine, 35*(3), 272–285.

This article details a quantitative study looking at the benefits of mindfulness-based stress reduction (MBSR) for improving affect and reducing depressive symptoms in gay men living with HIV. The study included 117 participants who were given questionnaires pre- and postintervention, as well as at 6 months follow-up. Results include: significant benefits of MBSR: at postintervention and 6 months follow-up, MBSR participants had significantly lower avoidance in IES and higher positive affect compared to controls. Participants with MBSR increased their mindfulness at two assessment periods (8 weeks and 6 months). Mindfulness was measured for these participants using the Toronto Mindfulness Scale (TMS), with the TMS subscales of curiosity and decentering.

Greason, P. B., & Cashwell, C. S. (2009). Mindfulness and counseling self-efficacy: The mediating role of attention and empathy. *Counselor Education and Supervision, 49*, 2–19.

This article was a quantitative study exploring the relationship between mindfulness and counseling self-efficacy. The authors also examined how attention and empathy might mediate counseling self-efficacy. There were 179 counseling master's-level and doctoral interns who completed measures of mindfulness, attention, empathy, and counseling self-efficacy. The hypothesis of the study—that mindfulness is a predictor of counseling self-efficacy—was confirmed by the results. Therefore, the authors asserted that mindfulness approaches should be integrated into counselor education, training, and supervision.

hold you steady and help you to focus your search for information. We strongly recommend that you write down your anchor questions and keep track of how they change during your search.

As you find more and more research and begin reading it, you will need to change your anchor from a question to a statement. You will need to put some kind of statement in writing that describes the purpose of your research. You might think of this as something like a thesis statement. It is a statement that anchors your search for literature. Importantly, this statement is meant to be changed. As you read and as you find more research, you can and should change this statement. Once again, we recommend that you keep track of how your statement changes over time. When you are ready to begin writing your literature review, it can be very helpful to see how your thoughts changed as you found more research, so it is good to have a journal of your thought process.

Let us take a look at anchor statements for stand-alone and preamble-to-research literature reviews. In a stand-alone literature review, a writer must have some sort of overall perspective or point of view that she is proposing. This perspective or point of view may not seem like an argument in the sense that the writer is proposing something new. Rather, the writer's argument in a stand-alone review of literature may read more like an overarching observation. Regardless, the argument or observation must be something that is supported by the literature that she includes in the literature review. See the excerpts and commentary in Table 7.2 for an illustration of how writers of stand-alone reviews of literature might state their arguments.

TABLE 7.2. Sample Arguments from Stand-Alone Literature Reviews
Text 1
Yet, despite these centrifugal restructurings, there remains a consistent need for and symbolism around the gayborhood (Grewal, 2008). It seems like an appropriate time, then, to ruminate on the place of this archetypical urban form (Brown, 2014, p. 358).
Commentary on Text 1
As you can see, Brown (2014) is writing a literature review on the gayborhood. His statements suggest that he intends to review literature that has explored the role that this space has had, currently has, and may have in the future. His field of study is geography, so, of course, we would imagine that his search for relevant literature begins with subfields of geography like cultural and critical geography. However, we would imagine that urban planning and queer studies might hold relevant literature for him as well.
Text 2
Much of the work I review here draws on Hall, Hart, and the concept of articulation quite directly, some more indirectly. While the concept thus runs through my entire review, I will examine the modalities of articulation by noting some of the different themes that critical geographers concerned with articulation—and related concepts—have elaborated in their work on race (Glassman, 2010, p. 507).
Commentary on Text 2
Glassman (2010) is writing a literature review on the treatment of articulation by critical geographers who study race. His statements specify critical geography as the field of interest, so we imagine that he would search for relevant literature in this field. However, we also imagine that he would look for relevant literature in sociology and ethnic studies to further address his focus on race. In both cases, we imagine that the writer may be summarizing and synthesizing literature from different fields.

The primary difference between the argument that is put forward in a stand-alone literature review and that of a preamble-to-research literature review would be the overall scope of the argument. A preamble-to-research literature review is going to move from the broader context to the narrower context much more quickly, because the review will be much shorter. A preamble-to-research literature review may also simply be more narrowly focused than a stand-alone literature review. See the excerpts and commentary in Table 7.3 for an illustration of how writers of preamble-to-research literature reviews might state their arguments.

If you articulate your anchor statement, you can return to it and evaluate each piece of literature in relation to it. In contrast, if your argument is only vaguely conceived in your mind, you have no point from which to determine relevance—truly, many things could be relevant. If you actually write your argument down, you can ask yourself, "How close or far is this literature in relation to my argument?" If explaining the connection between the literature and your argument would require more than a few sentences, it's probably too far away. Again, it is important to remember that the connection does not have to be one of agreement. You should be attentive to including points of view different from your own in your literature review. If you don't, your review will be challenged on the basis that it does not present a fair-minded picture of the context.

TABLE 7.3. Sample Arguments from Preamble-to-Research Literature Reviews

Text 1

In this paper, we examine how top-down and bottom-up sources of information each contribute to how speakers gesture during spontaneous narrative, and how such factors may influence one another. We begin by reviewing evidence for adaptation, which we find to be driven both top-down and bottom-up (Kuhlen, Galati, & Brennan, 2012, p. 19).

Commentary on Text 1

In Kuhlen, Galati, and Brennan (2012), the scope of the review of literature is limited to research on how top-down and bottom-up information affects speakers' adaptation.

Text 2

Relatively little research has been done on how victims cope with the experience of having been abused sexually as a child and whether or not CSA [childhood sexual abuse] influences a survivor's coping styles (Walker-Williams, van Eeden, & van der Merwe, 2012, p. 618).

Commentary on Text 2

In Walker-Williams, van Eeden, and van der Merwe (2012), the scope of the review of literature is limited to the ways that adult survivors of childhood sexual abuse cope with their experiences of abuse.

After a certain amount of research, it is important to move to writing about what you have found. However, moving to writing does not mean abandoning research. You should continue looking for literature as you write. In fact, as you write, you may have new ideas about key words for searches, or you may discover new literature through the references used in literature that you have already found.

DEVELOPING A POSITION STATEMENT FOR YOUR LITERATURE REVIEW

One of the first things you will need to decide and draft is a position statement, which may also be referred to as a statement of contribution, for your literature review. In academic writing, a position statement is usually a short paragraph that minimally includes two elements, the writer's argument and rationale. The argument is the part of the position statement that tells the readers where they are going if they read this literature review. It essentially tells readers what they will learn if they read this literature review. If you created an anchor statement, you have already started working on the argument. The rationale is the part of the position statement that tells the reader why following the argument is important.

Position statements are supposed to be directly and clearly stated. Readers should be able to locate your position statement easily and early in any academic text you write. They should be able to identify your primary argument and have a basic understanding of why your argument is meaningful within the context of your discipline. Position statements are concise but dense, meaning that they convey a lot of information in relatively few words. They are powerful in the sense that they establish your credibility and set your readers' expectations.

You will necessarily write and rewrite your position statement many times as you write your literature review, because as you write you will learn. Your initial ideas about how things fit together and what they mean will change, and those changes will need to be integrated into your position statement. So treat the writing of the position statement like aiming for a moving target and be willing to see it as a process rather than a product.

Across disciplines, position statements can be written in various ways, so be sure to notice how position statements within your field are typically articulated as you review your articles. However, in most disciplines, position statements are some variation on the following formula:

- Research does exist on X (past scholarship with often multiple in-text citations).
- But there is little information on Y (your topic of scholarship).
- This lack of information is potentially problematic for Z (persons or situations that may be affected by this absence of information).

Position statements typically appear in the beginning section of a paper. They are *not* usually the first paragraph of a paper, but they may be the second paragraph depending on the paper. They often follow one or more paragraphs that discuss past research. These paragraphs discussing past research are being used to set the stage for the delivery of the position statement. In many cases, the position statement may be the final paragraph of the beginning section of a paper, which means that it is the last paragraph a reader sees before the literature review (often the second section of a paper). Regardless of its location, the position statement clarifies the writer's position with regard to the topic and positions the reader to understand the literature review in a way that is aligned with the writer's argument. See the excerpt and commentary in Table 7.4 for a more detailed discussion.

In literature reviews, position statements develop a general context for the particular points you will make in your literature review. When articulating the argument and rationale, remember that this is not a personal position, so it is also important that you do not emotionally intensify

TABLE 7.4. Sample Position Statement

Text

[1]Given these statistics, counselors are likely to encounter clients (many of them women) who are taking antidepressants. [2]Yet as Schaefer and Wong-Wylie (2008) found in their Canadian study, counselors vary considerably in their attitudes, practices, and training regarding antidepressants. [3]Many bemoan the lack of clear guidelines on whether counseling alone, antidepressants alone, or a combination is optimal for treatment of depression. [4]Furthermore, the literature comparing the effectiveness of antidepressants and counseling for depression is vast, complex, and often contradictory. [5]And there is a paucity of concise and critical reviews of this literature, particularly from a counseling perspective (Hagen, Wong-Wylie, & Pijl-Zieber, 2010, p. 103).

Commentary

This position statement displays everything that we have just discussed. Sentence 1 clearly points to information (i.e., statistics) in a previous paragraph, so we know that this is not the first paragraph. Sentence 1 also proposes that this information (i.e., statistics on antidepressant use) affects a particular group of people (i.e., counselors), so we know to whom this topic is meaningful. Sentence 2 cites literature to support the idea that counselors are indeed affected by antidepressant use, sentence 3 elaborates on a particular need that counselors have with regard to antidepressant use, and sentence 4 refers to literature to further provide evidence for the problems that counselors have with antidepressant use. Sentences 2–4 further convince us that this topic is meaningful, especially to counselors. Sentence 5 points out that something is missing (i.e., "paucity") in the literature, which we understand that the writer intends to address with the literature review. Thus, as readers, we know where we are going (i.e., the argument) and why we are going there (i.e., the rationale).

your argument in any way and that you stick with a rational tone. (You may believe in the position on a personal level—in fact, we hope you do—but the position you are presenting is an academic one.) In Chapter 1, for instance, we talked about the concept of problematizing—treating a topic as if there is a problem that others have not seen or discussed enough—in academic writing. In your position statement, you will need to problematize other scholars' research in a way that is respectful. Successful position statements do not denigrate past work or create expectations that they cannot fill. For instance, don't set up a position statement that criticizes someone else's work or one that sets up a rationale that is not supported by your research.

OUTLINING YOUR LITERATURE REVIEW

Once you have a working draft of your position statement—and we stress the concept of draft because we do think it will change multiple times—you will need to plan the organization of your literature review. As we mentioned in Chapter 1, one of the strong general characteristics of academic writing is a high level of organization. Academic writing is typically organized on multiple levels: the macro-level (i.e., the sections and subsections of a text), the meso-level (i.e., the paragraphs within a section and/or subsection), and the micro-level (i.e., the sentences within a paragraph and the ideas within a single sentence). Achieving this type of multilevel organization requires planning before writing and often replanning while writing.

We are big proponents of using an outline to structure your literature review in planning before the writing stage for several reasons:

1. Outlines force you to organize the information you have collected into categories and to articulate the relationships you see between those categories, especially on the macro- and meso-levels.

2. Outlines help you see what you may be missing in your literature review.

3. Outlines remind you to stay true to your position statement all the way through the last sentence of your literature review.

4. Outlines save you time by helping you avoid going down a rabbit hole that has nothing to do with your literature review.

5. Outlines are quick and easy to design, and therefore quick and easy to send to peers and professors for feedback.

Do we have you convinced? Seriously, outlines are your best friend in the literature review process. To begin an outline for a stand-alone literature review, start with the basic organization listed below (we discuss outlines for preamble-to-research literature reviews in Chapter 8):

- Introduction: includes brief overview of topic selection, argument for topic selection, position statement of the literature review.
- Body: contains summaries, critiques, and syntheses of literature related to topic selection and argument of the literature review.
- Conclusion: revisits the introduction section through reminding the reader of the literature review topic and argument to draw conclusions about the literature reviewed in the body.

Now that you know the three major sections of the literature review, it is time to talk about length. Typically, the introduction and conclusion sections are about the same length, with the majority of the literature review spent in the body section. As students, sometimes you are given a certain page length for a literature review assignment, such as "Write a 20-page literature review." Let us say our topic is on the efficacy of antidepressants versus counseling to treat depression, to borrow the literature review topic used by Hagen, Wong-Wylie, and Pijl-Zieber (2010). You will likely write two to three pages of introduction and two to three pages of conclusion, leaving you with 14–16 pages for the body of the literature review. For those who like to crunch numbers and prefer even more structure, let's say your outline has three major sections of the body of the literature review and, "ta-da!," you know that you likely need to write approximately five pages for each of these three sections, more or less. See, outlines help you break down your ultimate writing of the literature review into more concrete goals.

Of course, as you begin writing, all of these page-length scenarios may not apply to what is needed based on the particular literature you are reviewing, but you can still see the literature review outline is a great place to start. Other times, you will not receive an assignment with a page length attached but will be writing a literature review that is of sufficient length to describe the literature in an area. In these cases, we suggest speaking with peers and professors to approximate a page length to get you started. Again, imposing structure on the literature review from the outset—even if you just know that the literature review chapter of your discipline's dissertations tend to be long—can help you nail down the outline and begin to set literature review writing goals.

Outlines come in many forms, from brief outlines to annotated outlines that are more descriptive. A good place to begin is with the brief outline. For a brief outline, the writer must consider all of the subtopics that he wishes to discuss about the general topic. Then he must organize those subtopics into sections and subsections. In the case of Hagen et al. (2010), the organizing structure on a macro-level includes six sections, and sections II–V (the body) include between two and six subsections:

I. Introduction

II. The comparable effectiveness of antidepressants and counseling

    A. Monotherapy for nonsevere depression

    B. Monotherapy for chronic or severe depression

III. Combination therapy: The more, the better?

    A. Nonsevere depression: Combination versus monotherapy

    B. Severe or chronic depression: Combination versus monotherapy

IV. Methodological limitations

    A. Limitations of systematic reviews and meta-analyses

    B. Issues with the measurement of depression

    C. Sampling issues

    D. Issues related to counseling interventions

    E. Lack of qualitative research

V. Pausing for thought: Other important considerations

    A. The placebo effect

    B. Trauma and depression

    C. Prevention of suicide

    D. Safety and side effects

    E. Cost issues

    F. The marketing of antidepressants

VI. Summary and implications

One of the tricky things in designing your outline is setting up an order for the review of subtopics within your literature review. In this case, subtopics refer to major areas of research *and* branches of research within those areas. For instance, you may have three major areas of past scholarship related to your topic that you are reviewing, and these three areas may contain different branches of research. Each major area represents a section of your text, and each branch represents a subsection. As a writer, you have to impose a sequential order on these three major areas and their branches, although there may not necessarily be an inherent order to guide you. For example, date of publication is a chronological order, but chronological order often means very little in academic research, because a topic may have been researched from several different perspectives by different researchers at the same chronological time. One solution is to, as you review the order of your outline, ask yourself what the relationships between the three major areas are. Is one major area more general? If so, that major area should be the first section of the body.

Once you have organized the major areas, you will need to repeat the process for the branches within each major area. Organizing branches may follow a general-to-specific order, but often that doesn't make sense because none of the branches is general. In this case, you might organize branches chronologically according to when research began on different branches. Of course, the development of research over time in the various branches may have been simultaneous, so you will necessarily include discussions of research about a specific branch in its specific subsection irrespective of its chronological date. The organization you select should be one that ultimately supports your argument by guiding your reader to accept the logic of your argument. See the subtopics representing major areas in the Hagen et al. (2010) literature review and the commentary that accompanies them in Table 7.5 for a discussion of their organizational strategy. Also, see the branches discussed for the different major areas from Hagen et al. (2010) and the commentary that accompanies them in Tables 7.6 and 7.7 for a discussion of their organizational pattern.

Each of the organizational and management strategies you have followed for collecting literature can prove very helpful when you are putting

TABLE 7.5. Sample Organization of Subtopics Representing Major Areas
Text
I. The comparable effectiveness of antidepressants and counseling
II. Combination therapy: The more, the better?
III. Methodological limitations
IV. Pausing for thought: Other important considerations
Commentary
There are four major areas within the body section that are organized moving from a first, more general subtopic to more specific considerations. Section I begins with literature that compares the general effectiveness of two types of treatment for depression. Section II moves to literature that looks at how those two types of treatment work in combination. Section III presumably discusses limitations of the types of studies that have been done to evaluate the effectiveness of the two types of treatment for depression. Section IV introduces other considerations that may have or would affect research on the two types of treatment for depression. From a general to specific perspective, this order seems logical because the readers' understanding of the topic is progressing from a wide-angle comparison of the two types of treatment to an increasingly more nuanced consideration of the issues affecting an understanding of the two types of treatment.

TABLE 7.6. Sample Organization of Branches Using Parallel Structure.
Text
II. The comparable effectiveness of antidepressants and counseling
A. Monotherapy for nonsevere depression
B. Monotherapy for chronic or severe depression
III. Combination therapy: The more, the better?
A. Nonsevere depression: Combination versus monotherapy
B. Severe or chronic depression: Combination versus monotherapy
Commentary
In section II, Hagen et al. (2010) discuss the branch focusing on nonsevere depression first and the branch focusing on chronic or severe depression second. They follow this same organizational pattern in section III. This is an example of parallel structure on a macro-level. In parallel structure, writers repeat patterns that they have previously used. The repetition of patterns helps readers to follow an argument without becoming confused because it simplifies the work their brains have to do with ordering and understanding information. Whenever possible, writers should use parallel structure at the macro-level of organization.

together the brief outline of the macro-structure of your literature review. Strategies such as creating category folders for articles or Excel spreadsheets of articles or annotated bibliographies are all ways that you discover the categories and patterns in the research that has been done. Your outline then reflects your unique perspective of how the puzzle pieces of the past fit together to form the current picture. You should view your outline as a working draft, as it is important to receive feedback on your outline and revise your outline as you review additional material. Be sure to provide anyone you ask for feedback with your position statement, as well as your outline, so that she can assess both in relation to one another. Some people like to outline by hand, and we suggest using a computer document ultimately so you can expand the document and even write in thoughts that will lay the foundations for sentences in future drafts. As you annotate and expand your outline more and more, be sure to look for ways to continue your argument by asking yourself, "How do these subheadings relate back to my original position statement in this literature review?"

WRITING THE INTRODUCTION OF YOUR LITERATURE REVIEW

You may wonder why you draft the position statement, which is one part of the introduction, and an outline of your entire literature review *before* you write the introduction. You may be thinking, "Isn't the introduction first? Why didn't they just tell me to start at the beginning?" A lot of people think this. That is, they think chronologically or sequentially. They imagine that the written text reflects the same order as the thought process behind the writing. They think that the introduction of an academic text is like the beginning of the writer's thought process, but the introduction actually represents thoughts the writer had *after* he had already worked out his entire thought process. In fact, the introduction is more like an invitation to something that has already happened. The reader is being invited to enter into a thought process that has already occurred and come to completion, so it is generally written after the writer has a clear idea of the entire thought process that will be covered in a text.

TABLE 7.7. Sample Organization of Branches Using General-to-Specific Pattern
Text
IV. Methodological limitations
A. Limitations of systematic reviews and meta-analyses
B. Issues with the measurement of depression
C. Sampling issues
D. Issues related to counseling interventions
E. Lack of qualitative research
V. Pausing for thought: Other important considerations
A. The placebo effect
B. Trauma and depression
C. Prevention of suicide
D. Safety and side effects
E. Cost issues
F. The marketing of antidepressants
Commentary
In these sections, Hagen et al. (2010) have followed a quasi-general-to-specific approach for organizing the branches. For example, item A of section IV focuses on general limitations, while items B–E focus on specific issues. It is possible that the order of the specific issues is related to how much literature the authors have on each issue (i.e., it could be in a most-to-least order). In section V, the ordering of the subsections is likely based on the grouping of similar considerations into a general-to-specific order. For example, item A is probably a group by itself. Items B and C are probably one group, with trauma and depression being more general than suicide. Item D is probably a group by itself. Items E and F are probably one group, with cost being a more general issue (or a more serious issue) than marketing.

Now, as you know, the position statement is drafted early in the writing process, but a position statement is not the same as an introduction. It is more like the "conclusion" of the introduction. The introduction has several functions that it must fulfill before the reader arrives at the position statement. For example, the introduction must hook the reader and draw her into the text. It must guide the reader to accept the logic of the position statement by providing information that supports that logic. And it must establish the credibility of the writer by demonstrating that she has done her homework. Then, once it arrives at the position statement, it must introduce the argument and the rationale that will be addressed by the rest of the text. After the position statement, the introduction needs to establish a vision for readers so that they will know where they are headed.

We like to think of the introduction as being made up of four parts on the meso-level: the hook, the bridge, the vision statement, and the position statement. You write the position statement first and likely many times over before you draft the hook, the bridge, and the purpose statement. Coming up with a hook and a bridge is like a backward design activity—you already know where you want to go (i.e., position statement), but you have to figure out the steps that you need to follow in order to get there. It helps to reflect on the following questions when you are trying to come up with a hook and a bridge:

- "How can I hook my reader and get him to see that my topic is an important *problem*?"
- "Once I hook the reader, what type of evidence do I need to provide in order to lead him from my hook to my position statement?"
- "How should I organize my evidence so that it leads logically to my position statement?"

Whereas the hook and the bridge are leading the reader to the position statement, the vision statement is telling them the path that they will follow after the position statement. The vision statement includes a purpose statement and a "road map." The purpose statement reminds your reader of your argument. We like purpose statements that are clear and concise and that literally include the word *purpose* in the sentence to guide the reader back to the argument for the importance of the literature review. Following the purpose statement, we encourage our students to write a "road map" sentence that spells out for the reader where you will go next. This actually brings us back to the importance of using outlines for your literature review writing. When you are writing from an outline, you can "see" what you will be writing about and tell the reader what is coming next in your paper. Let us take a look at how all of this happens in Table 7.8, using an excerpt from Hagen et al. (2010, pp. 102–103).

TABLE 7.8. Sample Introduction

Text

Paragraph 1

[1]Depression affects 9.5% of the U.S. population 18 years and older (NIMH, 2008), and women suffer depression at twice the rate of men (Antonuccio, Danton, DeNetsky, Greenbert, & Gordon, 1999; Nemeroff et al., 2003; Stoppard, 1999). [2]Worldwide depression rates have increased 1,000-fold since the emergence of selective serotonin reuptake inhibitor (SSRI) antidepressants 15 years ago (Currie, 2005), and the World Health Organization (WHO) has predicted that by 2020 depression will be the second leading source of global disability (WHO, 2007).

Paragraph 2

[3]Most persons with depression are treated by primary care physicians (Olfson, Marcus, Druss, Elinson, Tanielian, & Pineus, 2002), and 87 to 89 percent of U.S. physician visits for depression result in antidepressant prescriptions (Olfson et al.; Stafford, MacDonald, & Finkelstein, 2001). [4]The number of antidepressant prescriptions in Canada has increased exponentially, from 3.2 million in 1981 to 14.5 million in 2000 (Hemels, Koren, & Einarson, 2002), and the percentage of persons treated for depression with antidepressants in the U.S. jumped from 37.3% in 1987 to 74.5% in 1997 (Olfson et al.). [5]Just as women are diagnosed with depression at twice the rate of men, they are given antidepressants at twice the rate (Munoz, Hollon, McGrath, Rehm, & VandenBos, 1994). [6]Canadian statistics show that one in five women in the province of British Columbia was taking one or more SSRIs between 2002 and 2003 (Currie, 2005).

Paragraph 3

[7]Given these statistics, counselors are likely to encounter clients (many of them women) who are taking antidepressants. [8]Yet as Schaefer and Wong-Wylie (2008) found in their Canadian study, counselors vary considerably in their attitudes, practices, and training regarding antidepressants. [9]Many bemoan the lack of clear guidelines on whether counseling alone, antidepressants alone, or a combination is optimal for treatment of depression. [10]Furthermore, the literature comparing the effectiveness of antidepressants and counseling for depression is vast, complex, and often contradictory. [11]And there is a paucity of concise and critical reviews of this literature, particularly from a counseling perspective.

Paragraph 4

[12]Therefore, the purpose of this paper is to critique the literature on the comparable effectiveness of counseling and antidepressants for treating depression in adults. [13]Given the 100+ research studies on this topic, this review is limited to *systematic reviews* and *meta-analyses* of studies published in the last 20 years (1987 onward). [14]We also review issues that influence an understanding of the literature and conclude with recommendations for counseling practice.

(continued)

TABLE 7.8. *(continued)*

Commentary

Overall

The first paragraph provides the hook, the second functions as a bridge, the third is the position statement, and the fourth is the vision statement. Just to be clear, not all introductions are four paragraphs. Some introductions can accomplish the functions of each part in less than three paragraphs, and some require more than three paragraphs.

Paragraph 1

Paragraph 1 hooks the reader by problematizing depression through the use of shocking facts that should provoke concern in the reader. We learn quickly that 9.5% of the adult U.S. population is depressed, worldwide depression rates are 1,000 times higher than they were 15 years ago, and depression is predicted to be a primary cause of global disability by 2020. We are inclined to believe these facts because the writer has referred to six different reputable sources in the paragraph.

Paragraph 2

Now that we are hooked by our concern about the problem of depression, paragraph 2 establishes a bridge between the general problem of depression to the more specific problem of antidepressants. In the second paragraph, we are again provided with facts from reputable sources that are designed to convince us that antidepressant use is widespread, and, of course, the implication is that this is because depression is widespread.

Paragraph 3

By the time we reach paragraph 3, we are or should be persuaded that depression is a serious problem that has led to the widespread use of antidepressants, which sets us up perfectly for the writer's delivery of the position statement. Now, we just need to know why this matters (rationale) and what the writer intends to do (argument). Paragraph 3 delivers this information by explaining that these topics are especially meaningful for counselors because they treat people with depression (i.e., rationale) and that relatively little is known about the effectiveness of counseling versus antidepressants for the treatment of depression (i.e., argument).

Paragraph 4

Paragraph 4 leads us from the position statement into the rest of the paper by establishing a clear vision of where we are going. We are told exactly what the purpose of the paper is in sentence 12. We are provided a road map that lets us know the general topics—systematic reviews, meta-analyses, issues that influence an understanding of the literature, and recommendations for counseling practice—that will be covered in the paper.

> **BOX 7.4. Meso-Level Organization of the Introduction**
>
> I. Introduction
>   1. Hook
>   2. Bridge
>   3. Position Statement
>   a. Rationale
>   b. Argument
>   4. Vision Statement
>   a. Purpose
>   b. Road Map

As we mentioned before, the length of the introduction really is dependent on your overall goal for your literature review and whether or not you have been given a fixed page limit. Typically, we suggest that the introduction should range from about 10 to 20% of your overall literature review length. Overall, the introduction serves as the main organizer of your literature review. You reference the major ideas and constructs you will discuss in your literature review related to past scholarship. See Box 7.4 for a general outline of the Introduction at the meso-level and use Practice Exercise 7.1 to analyze a sample introduction from a literature review in your field.

PRACTICE EXERCISE 7.1. Analyzing Introductions in Your Field

Select a review of literature research article in your field. Read only the introduction. Identify the following parts of the introduction. Remember that these parts are not always neatly accomplished in one paragraph or one sentence. For example, sometimes the bridge may span over several paragraphs.

- Hook
- Bridge
- Position statement
  - Rationale
  - Argument
- Vision statement
  - Purpose
  - Road map

WRITING THE BODY OF THE LITERATURE REVIEW

By the time you have arrived at the midsection of your literature review, you should congratulate yourself! You have engaged in a good deal of work, you understand your topic a little more, and possibly you even are more interested in the topic of your literature review! Roll up your sleeves and check the outline you have for the body of your literature review. This outline will guide your first steps. You will also draw upon the organizing tools you set up when initially searching the literature, from any notes you jotted down during your review of past scholarship to your annotated bibliography.

Writing within Each Subtopic

The outline really becomes your best friend in getting the nitty-gritty progression of ideas within each subsection. Your brief outline of the macro-structure can become increasingly longer and more detailed as you decide the meso-level structure of how you will organize the paragraphs within each subsection. You have already seen the meso-level structure of the introduction in the previous section. Meso-level organization follows the same basic principles as macro-level organization. You have to establish an order of presentation that supports the argument you are building, and whenever possible that order should be from general to specific. See Box 7.5 from Hagen et al. (2010) as an example of meso-level organization and notice the use of parallel structure at the meso-level, as well as the macro-level.

It is important to note that subsections may have several paragraphs, or they may just be one paragraph. If a subsection is only one paragraph, then the organization you need to consider is at the micro-level of structure, because you are considering how the sentences and ideas are ordered within the paragraph. In general, writers do not usually outline paragraphs at the micro-level, because it is a sentence-by-sentence structure, but you could

---

BOX 7.5. Meso-Level Structure

I. The comparable effectiveness of antidepressants and counseling

  A. Monotherapy for nonsevere depression

    1. Summary of findings for effectiveness of using just antidepressants or just counseling as treatment

    2. Suggestions resulting from findings

  B. Monotherapy for chronic or severe depression

    1. Summary of findings for effectiveness of using just antidepressants or just counseling as treatment

if you were struggling to connect phrases and ideas. It can be very helpful to create reverse outlines of other writers' paragraphs to figure out the organization strategies that they followed at the micro-level. In a reverse outline, you analyze each sentence of a paragraph to figure out the purpose the writer was trying to achieve with each sentence in order to understand the overall structure of the paragraph. Reverse outlines are very good for helping you understand the relationship between purpose and structure. See Table 7.9 for an example of a reverse outline of a one-paragraph section from Hagen et al. (2010, p. 104).

Critiquing and Synthesizing Literature

As we have alluded to throughout this chapter, a literature review is not just a summary. Rather, a literature review is a synthesis. A synthesis implies that the writer has reviewed multiple sources and is presenting a unique

TABLE 7.9. Using Reverse Outlines for Understanding Micro-Level Structure
B. Monotherapy for chronic or severe depression
1. Summary of findings for effectiveness of using just antidepressants or just counseling as treatment
Text
Monotherapy for Chronic or Severe Depression
[1]Fewer studies have compared antidepressant and counseling monotherapy for the treatment of adults with chronic or severe depression, and the conclusions are less consistent than for studies of nonsevere depression. [2]Three reviews (Hollon, Thase, & Markowitz, 2002; Jacobson & Hollon, 1996; Spencer & Nashelsky, 2005) and one meta-analysis (deRubeis, Gelfand, Tang, & Simons, 1999) have concluded that counseling alone is as effective as antidepressants alone for severe or chronic depression, although two other reviews reached the opposite conclusion (Amow & Constantino, 2003; Michalak & Lam, 2002). [3]Thus, the comparable effectiveness of either monotherapy for chronic or severe depression is less clear and may be subject to researcher bias.
Reverse Outline
What is the purpose of each sentence?
Sentence 1: Express the general idea that findings are few and inconsistent.
Sentence 2: Support the general idea by enumerating the relatively small number of studies on this topic and the contrasting nature of their findings.
Sentence 3: Offer an observation that is a logical conclusion based on the information provided in sentence 2. This observation supports the writers' overall position (i.e., there is insufficient research on the general topic of the article).

perspective on how those sources merge with one another in creating a picture that cannot be created by just a few sources. When writing a stand-alone literature review, you are finding and bringing together pieces of a puzzle; however, the picture they will form is determined by you. This is why decision making plays such a crucial role in literature reviews.

When writing a literature review, you are summarizing, but you are doing so with the purpose of finding connections, contradictions, and implications between different studies. You are also summarizing with the purpose of finding problems or gaps in the research that has been done. While the initial critique of literature begins as you are searching for and organizing literature using various management tools, it is natural that, as you learn more and more about a topic, you understand the literature you have read related to your topic further and can therefore engage in a more in-depth critique of the literature you have selected to review.

As you plan and outline the macro-structure of your literature review, you ask yourself how more general ideas fit together, and you synthesize your ideas by imposing an organizational structure that reflects your argument. As you plan the meso-structure of each section or subsection, you have to consider all of the sources that you plan to use in that section. You have to know the main ideas and findings of each, and your understanding of those must be accurate. In addition, you must have some ideas about how the ideas and findings of these sources fit together. When considering the relationships between different studies, it may be helpful to ask yourself the following questions:

- Do they support each other?
- Do they contradict each other?
- Do the ideas or findings of one source add to or explain the ideas or findings of another?
- Do the ideas and findings of multiple sources replicate each other, or are they inconsistent?

At the meso-level, you also have to consider the manner in which the studies were done. After all, the findings of any study may be fundamentally flawed or suspect if the manner in which they were obtained is improper or lacking in some way. Therefore, methodological or interpretative critiques are part of what you should consider when you are summarizing articles in preparation for writing. Methodological critiques are observations on how researchers' choices in their studies may have influenced their findings. For example, a methodological critique might be that the number of participants was quite small or unbalanced in some way. Interpretative critiques are observations on how researchers interpreted or explained their findings. For example, you may find that a researcher's interpretation of her findings depends on too many assumptions or is simply not reasonable considering the data. You may remember that Lauren prefers annotated bibliographies that include summary + reflection + connection. If you have created this type of annotated bibliography when you were gathering sources, your reflection commentary would include critiques, and your connection commentary would include thoughts on the intersections between different studies.

Writing the body of your literature review is generally a writing-to-learn experience, meaning that you usually discover connections and critiques while you write that you had not considered before writing. These discoveries are wonderful and should be incorporated. However, you have to be mindful of how new ideas affect your argument and your macro-structure. The principle of relevance applies to writing as well as gathering research. Everything has to be related to your argument and organized in such a way that your argument seems logical to the reader. Sometimes novice writers discover new ideas and go crazy writing about those ideas, but they forget to go back and change their introduction and macro-structure to line up with these new ideas. The result, in those cases, is a road to nowhere. Readers wind up confused and frustrated, and they may question the writer's credibility.

We cannot stress enough the importance of rereading and rewriting. In this case, we mean rereading your own work. Everything flows from your introduction, so it is extremely important to reread your literature review as you write it, from the beginning to wherever you are. If your literature review is relatively short (10–20) pages, this is easy to do. You should simply reread what you have written every time you sit down to work on your review, even if you leave it for only a few hours. As you do this rereading, you should constantly be imagining how your reader would be responding to the development of your argument. If you notice gaps in your argument, you need to fix those before you move on with your writing. Yes, this might slow you down, but ultimately it will result in a better literature review. If you see organization issues or style issues, fix those as you are doing this rereading. Every time you reread—and that should be multiple times if you do it every time you work on your review—you have the opportunity to make it a little bit better. You may find, as Lauren recalls in Box 7.6, that sometimes you have to basically "blow up" what you have done and start over to make it better. Don't be afraid to do this—it might actually make the rest of your writing easier!

Of course, the longer the text you are writing is, the harder it is to conceive of starting over or making changes that will drastically alter the argument. This is probably why many novice writers try so hard to make arguments work even when they know that they do not have enough evidence or the right kind of evidence for the argument. Rereading a dissertation from the beginning to the point at which you left off every time you come back to your writing is difficult, if not impossible at some point. Reverse outlining can help in these cases. We explained how to use reverse outlining earlier in this chapter for understanding other writers' micro-level

BOX 7.6. Fifteen Pages in the Wrong Direction Is Not Time Wasted

It was really hard for me to write my dissertation—I mean *really* hard. I just couldn't get my rhythm with how to do it, because I'm just a person who needs large chunks of time (I now know that the chunks have to be at least 4 hours) to really get into the writing and make progress. That kind of time is really hard to find when you are teaching full time, settling into a new living-together arrangement after living alone for many years, and planning a wedding. It doesn't help when you are also a perfectionist who procrastinates. It was essentially a perfect storm situation. Nonetheless, it had to get done. Vacations became some of the only times when I could get things going, so for better or for worse, no matter where we went, I took everything I needed to write, and sometimes I actually did it. I still remember one time when I had spent 2 full days of what was supposed to be a beach vacation inside writing one of the chapters of my dissertation. (I did sit in front of the window so that I could see the beach.) It was one of the first times that I had made any real progress with getting my ideas out and down on paper. I really thought I was getting somewhere. It is my habit to reread as I write any time I leave my writing or come back to it or any time I am just trying to think of where to go next. Sometimes I even stop writing and use reverse outlining of what I have written to be sure that I understand the argument as I have presented it thus far so that I will know where to go. Toward the end of the second day, I realized through my rereading and reverse outlining that where I was headed wasn't where I needed to go. And, to make matters worse, nothing I had done was really helpful for where I needed to go. In other words, I basically needed to start over. Now, that could have caused a complete shutdown in my process, but I had actually experienced situations like this before (although not any that involved so many pages). I knew from past experience that writing in the wrong direction could sometimes be exactly what I needed to know in order to find the right direction, so I didn't consider the time wasted. I knew that even though I might not be able to use any of those pages as I had written them, the time spent articulating and connecting ideas had actually prepared me for what I needed to do. I also knew that it was likely that I had been in some way rehearsing things that I would, in fact, say in later writing or in a different way. Of course, even knowing all of these things, I didn't delete what I had written or anything crazy like that. I opened a new document and pasted all of it in but started writing again from the beginning, looking at what I had pasted in from time to time for inspiration. Eventually, when I had written enough to compensate for the pain of deletion, I did delete what I had pasted in, but I never deleted it in my draft documents. I always kept any writing I did in the right direction or the wrong direction simply because I did find that sometimes I wanted to remember the way I phrased something in a text I had previously written, or I wanted to remind myself of some idea that I had expressed.

—Lauren

structure. However, you can use an informal type of reverse outlining to keep up with your own meso- and micro-level organization.

The way that Lauren does this is by rereading what she has written with a pad of paper and pen in hand. She "takes notes" on what she has written, as if she were reading it for the purpose of taking notes. By doing this, she is trying to see whether she is able to take notes easily in an organized way. If she can, then she feels that it is likely that the organizational structure she used in the text she has written is logical and the connections are clear. If she notices that as a note taker she is struggling with the relationships between ideas or feeling like some information is out of order, then she knows as a writer that she needs to go back and make some changes to her written text. Once she makes those changes, she "takes notes" again to be sure that she has eliminated whatever problems she saw the first time and not created any more problems.

When you are writing a long text, these informal reverse-outlining notes are useful, helping you to keep track of what you have already discussed and where you discussed specific things in your text. This can save you time, because you don't have to hunt through pages and pages to double-check your information. You can also easily reread informal reverse-outline notes every time you start working on your text. They can quickly immerse you in the world of your argument, reacquainting you with your argument and reorienting you to where you need to go next.

WRITING THE FINAL SECTION OF THE LITERATURE REVIEW

Once you have arrived at the conclusion of your stand-alone literature review (remember, preamble-to-research literature reviews are discussed in Chapter 8), you will need to summarize some of the overall commonalities, contradictions, and other "surprises" you found within the literature base on your topic. In the Hagen et al. (2010) literature review, their final section is formally labeled "Summary and Implications," and it includes implications for counselors based on the scholarship they reviewed. See Table 7.10 for a list of the paragraphs included in their "Summary and Implications" and a discussion of how these paragraphs are organized.

A different pattern may be used when the final section of the literature review is leading toward your research question, such as in dissertation research. In this instance, the entire literature review itself is a contextualization of your research question, so your final section returns to your research question again as a logical outgrowth of your review of past scholarship.

Regardless of the pattern used in the summary section, in terms of the length of the literature review, we again think a good rule of thumb is for the introduction and the final section of the literature review to approximate the same length—10–20% of the overall length.

TABLE 7.10. Sample Organization for a Conclusion

Text

I. Summary and Implications
  1. Overall Summary of Comparison of Two Treatments for Depression
  2. Overall Critique of Limitations with Existing Literature
  3. Introduction of First Logical Implication of This Review for Counselors
  4. Introduction of Second Logical Implication of This Review for Counselors
  5. Introduction of Third Logical Implication of This Review for Counselors

Commentary

Each cardinal number (1–5) represents one paragraph in the text. You can see how each paragraph logically builds on the next. The first paragraph reminds the reader of the topics that have been the subject of the review and the facts that the writers have established about those topics. The second paragraph reminds the reader of the writers' argument (i.e., the problem the writer has found with the existing literature). The third through fifth paragraphs articulate the primary takeaways that the writers believe this review has for counselors, who were an important part of the writers' original rationale for writing this literature review. Thus the writers bring the journey of their review to completion by providing observations based on analysis of literature that are relevant to their original argument and rationale.

CONTINUING THE HUNT FOR LITERATURE WHILE YOU WRITE

We mentioned in our previous discussion of hunting and gathering literature that the search does not end when you begin writing; however, the search for literature does change. As you plan and write your literature review, you understand your topic and your overall focus more; and, as you understand your topic and focus more, you realize subtopics that you may have overlooked or not thought of when you were conducting your original search for literature. When you have these realizations, you will need to return to the hunt, but, of course, this time you will know more specifically what you are trying to find. You may also realize as you write that you have overemphasized certain subtopics simply because you found more literature on them. In this case, you will probably need to cut back on those areas and look for more literature on other areas. It is natural if you feel frustrated in these instances. However, this is an integral aspect of academic writing related to the literature review. You simply cannot complete your review of all relevant scholarship before you write your literature review because writing a literature review is one of the ways that you actually learn the literature. You are immersed in it while you write, and that immersion helps you to see patterns and gaps that can only be seen when a person has really engaged deeply with a topic. So try not to see returning to the hunt as a backward step in the writing process; it's actually a forward step because it means that your knowledge about your topic has actually increased.

CHAPTER SUMMARY AND REMINDERS

In this chapter, we talked about how to search, organize, and write the literature review. Along the way, we discussed how to refine your keyword searches and stay on track with literature that is most relevant to your topic, and how to use organizing strategies such as outlines and annotated bibliographies to help you with the principle of relevance. We also reviewed the vital importance of developing a strong argument and tracking that argument throughout the three sections of the literature review—the introduction, body, and summary. See Summary Table 7.1 for awareness and action reminders.

SUMMARY TABLE 7.1. AWARENESS AND ACTION REMINDERS	
Be aware . . .	Take action . . .
Literature reviews establish your credibility as a researcher, and they help readers to accept your research questions as logical next steps in the development of literature on your topic.	Look for inspirational voices in the texts you read.
New ideas are often born from and through writing literature reviews.	Invite your personal curiosity to be part of your academic voice.
Searching for literature requires time, patience, and determination.	Organize articles into folders that represent categories as you find them and be sure to name articles in a way that makes it easy for you to know what the article is about.
Academic writing is a series of strategic but predictable moves.	Articulate your argument as a statement or question in writing as early as possible and evaluate the relevance of the literature you find in relation to the written version of your argument.
When you are writing to learn, as is often the case in literature reviews, position statements need to be evaluated and rewritten on a regular basis.	Draft a position statement and an outline to help you figure out what you want to say and how to best use the literature to support your position.

CHAPTER 8

The Writing Formula for Empirical Academic Writing

In previous chapters, we have discussed academic writing related to stand-alone literature reviews, and we have touched on how to write literature reviews that are designed to lead into a study you have conducted. In this chapter, we discuss the major sections typical of academic writing related to empirical work. For this book, *empirical academic writing* refers to writing moves you use within the Method, Results, and Discussion sections of your dissertation or other study.

Our **awareness focus** for this chapter is to help you to understand that there are specific ways in which you describe your literature review and method, report your results, and discuss your findings in these standard sections in your discipline's CoP. The **action focus** for this chapter is to help you to learn both the commonalities in empirical academic writing across disciplines and the unique ways that you write these standard sections within your CoP.

UNDERSTANDING THE PURPOSE OF STANDARD SECTIONS IN EMPIRICAL WRITING

Remember the first time you read an empirical article in your discipline? You might not remember the topic, but you may remember how it felt to begin reading empirical studies in journals for the first time and realize that there are standard sections. You probably were feeling fine reading through the literature review, and then, bam! The Method section probably felt like reading an entirely different language. Reading the Results section probably did not feel much easier. Then, getting to the Discussion section probably felt like a relief, as it decoded what the Method and Results sections were describing in somewhat of a summary form. The truth is that until you have taken your research-based courses, reading the Method and Results sections will likely continue to be like reading a different language. Even after you have these research-based classes under your belt, it may still feel that way when you are reading about a new methodology, and likewise a new way of reporting results.

Regardless, in this book we are concerned with how you write; and, if you are going to engage in any type of research activity, it is likely you will be called upon to know how to write these sections. Right now, we want to review the purpose of each of these sections before we dive in more deeply to describe what should be included. As you have learned already, the literature review of your study has certain set components. Your Method section (sometimes called a Methodology or Methods section) describes for the reader how you went about doing your study—basically, what the study procedures were from beginning to end. Your Results section (sometimes called a Findings section) describes the results of the data analysis in which you engaged. Your Discussion section describes how your results are similar to or different from previous research, as well as the implications and limitations of your study.

As we discuss empirical writing in this chapter, keep in mind that we are describing the general conventions you can follow. It is important to learn these general guidelines, hone your skills in these areas, and know that you may later deviate from these guidelines because your study demands a different presentation strategy. So there is a balance between knowing the conventions of empirical writing and not holding so tightly to these conventions that your organization becomes boring and formulaic. To get started in learning these conventions, let's review what might be different for a literature review for your study (i.e., a preamble-to-research literature review, as we called it in Chapter 7) versus a stand-alone literature review.

WRITING A LITERATURE REVIEW FOR A STUDY

One of the first differences in writing a literature review for a study, as compared to writing a stand-alone literature review, is the length. In a stand-alone literature review, your only goal is to write a literature review; so you have the luxury (although it might not feel like it) of using your entire manuscript length for this purpose. In writing a literature review for your study, there is a very specific goal: to provide evidence from previous literature for the importance of your study. This is where identifying the gap in your field related to your study topic, defining constructs, and many of the other tips for writing literature reviews come into play, as discussed in Chapter 7. You will necessarily have to make decisions about the length of your literature review that supports your study, and your overarching guide is answering this question:

What are the most salient components of previous literature related to your study topic that provide evidence for the need for your study?

In terms of length, many journals will have a set page limit for manuscripts, while thesis dissertation projects rarely have a page limit. If there is a page limit, you can use the rule of 25% to guide your writing—as in setting aside 25% of your manuscript for each of the following four sections: (1) Literature Review, (2) Method, (3) Results, and (4) Discussion sections. This is just a general rule for you to follow, and depending on the type of research approach you use, you may need to shift these percentages. For instance, in qualitative and mixed-methods studies, literature reviews may be the shortest sections, as there is a need for more space to describe the Method, Results, and Discussion sections, whereas in quantitative studies, the literature reviews tend to be longer, as tables and figures can be used in the Results section to concisely illustrate the data for the reader. In addition, the length of literature reviews in empirical academic writing can vary depending on your particular discipline, so you want to get intimately familiar with what the standards are for journals and thesis or dissertation projects in your field or department. Take a look at Practice Exercise 8.1 to explore how to write literature reviews for empirical studies.

PRACTICE EXERCISE 8.1. Writing Literature Reviews for Empirical Studies

Select three empirical articles, theses, or dissertations in your field. Read these articles and notice the following:

- What is the overall length of the literature review compared to the total manuscript length?
- What specific organizers (e.g., subheadings) do the authors use within their literature review?
- How do the authors transition to the Method section?

There is also the transition to the subsequent Method section. Often, at the end of the literature in empirical academic writing, scholars place their research question as the very last sentence as a way to bridge the Literature Review and Method sections. Anneliese does exactly this in the transition from her literature review to her Method section:

> The specific research question guiding the study was, how do trans youth describe the supports of and the challenges to their daily lived experiences of resilience? (Singh, Meng, & Hansen, 2014, p. 210)

In another example, the mixed-methods study by Theron, Lievenberg, and Malindi (2014), the authors conclude their literature review by using a transition signifying that the authors are expressing a result, language related to the goal of the study, and a statement of the research question:

> Thus, the aim of this article is to investigate whether, and how, schooling experiences that are respectful of child rights encourage youth resilience. We confine our focus to school experiences that are respectful of child rights because all participants in this study were school-going, because they commented directly on their experiences of school environments as a key focus of the study, and because schooling has the potential to nurture resilience (Luthar, 2006; Miller & Daniel, 2007). Our investigation was guided by the following questions: To what extent do rights-based school environments encourage youth resilience, and how do school environments that are respectful of youths promote positive youth adjustment? (p. 255)

Read Box 8.1 to see how Lauren approaches writing the literature review section.

WRITING THE METHOD SECTION

By the time you are ready to write a Method section, you should be well versed in how to engage in academic writing in general. For instance, by this point, you have learned that academic writing language is not speaking language but, rather, a formal endeavor that follows certain rules and organization strategies. You can think of the Method section similarly. Many of the Method sections in social and behavioral sciences involve human participants, so you will need to describe the overall procedure of

---

BOX 8.1. First-Person Narrative: Writing the Literature Review Section

My personal struggle with any literature review is that at some point, I see everything as connected. I have whatever is the opposite of tunnel vision. The more literature I find, the more I feel uncertain about how to situate my research question. The way I get around this uncertainty is to take a moment to reassess what I have and really ask myself if I am being perfectionistic about getting every single article on a subject. I ask myself, "If I were reading an argument about this research question, what would I need to know as a reader in order to accept the research question?"

—*Lauren*

how you interacted with participants, recruited (or sampled) participants, and demographic information about your participants. You will also need to provide information about the research setting and how you collected and analyzed data, including whether you used a qualitative, quantitative, or mixed-methods approach. Depending on which of these three research approaches you use, there will be specific information important to include. For instance, empirical academic writing for a qualitative study will necessarily include the type of research tradition you used (e.g., grounded theory, phenomenology), whereas a quantitative study will include the types of instruments or measures you used and their related validity and reliability information. When writing the Method section of a mixed-methods study, you will include all of the above and, importantly, the specific ways and timing of how you "mixed" the data (e.g., were qualitative data collected before quantitative data? Were the qualitative and quantitative data analyzed simultaneously or at different time intervals?). The overall essential components of a Method section, therefore, include the following subcategories (or subheadings) within the Method section:

- Description of research approach.
- Participant demographic information.
- Study procedure.
- Study instruments.
- Data collection and data analysis.

Sometimes these sections may be collapsed together (e.g., Participants and Procedure) or named differently (e.g., Ethics instead of Procedure), but, regardless, these subcategories are placed somewhere within the Method section. These subcategories are typically ordered in a chronological manner, moving from describing your research approach to who your participants are, how participants were recruited and protected, instruments used, and how data were collected and analyzed. However, your discipline may have unique ways of organizing these. In addition to the order of these sections varying across disciplines, the amount of information provided in each of the above sections can vary as well. For instance, a qualitative study in education may have a longer description of the research approach than a qualitative study in public health. So be sure to have a few exemplar articles in your discipline available across research approaches so you can study what those discipline-specific distinctions are.

Description of Research Approach

Your first task in the Method section is to tell your reader about the research approach you selected for your study. This type of empirical academic writing describes the qualitative, quantitative, or mixed-methods approach in detail. When describing a qualitative study, you will describe the research tradition you used and typically include information about the scholars who have developed these approaches. For example, in one of Anneliese's phenomenological studies, she describes for the reader not only what phenomenology is, but also one of the significant scholars who developed the phenomenological approach she is using:

> The selected phenomenological approaches allowed us (one counselor educator and two master's-level counseling students) to explore the essence and meaning of the supports of and challenges to resilience for trans youth participants (Hays & Singh, 2012; Moustakas, 1994). In addition, phenomenology allowed us to seek a deep structural understanding of the daily lived experiences of the resilience of trans youth participants. The theoretical framework of the study was based on Freire's (1971) liberation theology, including the tenets of anti-oppression and *conscientization* (i.e., consciousness raising). We also used tenets from feminist theory (Worrel & Remer, 2003)—specifically, "the personal is political" and valuation of sociopolitical identities—to develop research activities that were focused on empowerment. (Singh et al., 2014, p. 210)

Empirical academic writing in quantitative studies also describes the overall research approach; however, these descriptions are often much more brief.

Quantitative studies do not include a detailed description of the research approach, but instead describe the context of the study and the types of instruments used without as much description of the statistical method itself, such as this study by Goldblum and colleagues (2012):

> [This study] was a multiphase, multiyear project that culminated in a statewide survey of trans people that sought to identify the social and environmental risk factors associated with HIV and other health consequences in this population, and to ascertain how trans people access medical and mental health services (Bradford, Reisner, Honnold, & Xavier, in press; Bradford, Xavier, Hendricks, Rivers, & Honnold, 2007). Construction of the survey questionnaire was informed by an earlier phase of THIS, which collected qualitative data from focus groups of trans individuals (Bradford et al., 2007). The model informing the survey proposed that the social stigma of being trans and its manifestations (e.g., discrimination, violence) are the root cause of poor somatic and mental health outcomes, including HIV-positive serostatus, substance abuse, and suicidal ideation and attempts (Bradford et al., 2007). (p. 470)

In mixed-methods studies, the description of the research approach includes the study aim and the particular type of mixed-methods research approach, such as this mixed-methods study by Theron et al. (2014):

The overall aim of this study was to understand the formal service and informal pathways that encouraged youth resilience in high-risk contexts. For the purposes of this article, we report only the South African data. We employed an explanatory mixed-methods design to generate and interpret data (Creswell, 2009). (p. 255)

In the three previous examples, you can see how the length of the research description varies by the research approach and by disciplines.

Participant Demographic Information

This section may seem like a simple section—you report the demographics of your study participants. However, we often see that authors omit important information in this section. By the time you write your participant demographic information section, you should have already carefully contemplated who was included in and who was excluded from your study. Based on your study topic, you may elect to share more or less demographic information about your study. In Anneliese's study of transgender youth resilience, the most important demographic information was the gender identity, racial/ethnic identity, and current educational level. She also described the study sampling criteria, as in her qualitative study below:

The researchers used purposeful sampling to recruit participants over a 3-month period (Creswell, 2007). The criteria for participants in the study included the following: (a) between the ages of 15 and 25 years old and (b) identify as trans. There were 19 participants in the study and their mean age was 22 years. Thirteen participants were White, three were multiracial, two were African American, and one was Asian American/Pacific Islander. Seven participants were college graduates, seven were currently enrolled in college, one had earned an associate's degree, and two were high school graduates. One participant withdrew from college for medical reasons, and a second reported having dropped out of college. (Singh et al., 2014, p. 210)

Study Procedure, Including Participant Recruitment and Informed Consent

This section is essentially an overview of your study activities. The section is commonly called "Procedure" or "Study Procedure" and begins with the process of how you interacted with participants. We encourage you to also include informed consent procedures within the study. For instance, a procedure section typically begins with the geographic region where the study was conducted (e.g., general region such as "the southeastern U.S.," "an urban setting," "South Africa"). Next, you can provide a brief mention of securing institutional review board (IRB) approval and anything notable about that process. Following this is information about participant recruitment. The manner in which participants were sampled (e.g., electronic mailing lists, paper flyers, social media) is also included. In the Theron et al. (2014) mixed-methods article, the authors do not list "Procedure," instead titling this section "Contextualization."

> Bethlehem and Qwa, located in the Thabo Mofutsanyana District, Eastern Free State, South Africa, were our research sites. Bethlehem is a small rural town, while Qwa is a former rural homeland designated for the Basotho people. Together, these sites are characterized by risks to resilience, including extreme poverty and unemployment, poor infrastructure (including poor school facilities), marginal living conditions and services, crime and HIV & AIDS-related challenges (Heunis, Engelbrecht, Kigozi, Pienaar, & Van Rensburg, 2009). All of the aforementioned factors potentially compromise children's rights. Notwithstanding these risks, some youths have adjusted well. (p. 254)

Study Instruments

Study instruments also vary by type of research approach. In a qualitative study, the study instruments often include the researchers themselves, as their positionality is described in relation to the study topic, as in Anneliese's qualitative study:

> RESEARCHERS AS INSTRUMENTS
>
> We identified our assumptions and biases about the topic prior to engaging in the research process. Before submitting our research proposal to the institutional review board, the first and second author met to bracket these biases. The first author self-identified as a South Asian queer woman and had engaged in previous qualitative studies of trans people's resilience. Therefore, her assumptions about the topic were grounded in these studies and included a bias that all trans people are resilient in some manner. (Singh & McKleroy, 2011, p. 36)

Study instruments in qualitative studies can also include any demographic surveys used or media-based instruments (e.g., participant photography, participant journals), whereas in quantitative studies, the study instruments very narrowly describe surveys used and whether there is any reliability and validity information. In the Goldblum et al. (2012) quantitative study, the authors are using a self-reported, unvalidated survey; however, they still describe not only the overarching sections of the survey but also the type of information the survey was seeking from participants:

> In-school GBV [gender-based victimization]. School-based victimization was assessed by a series of questions. First, participants were asked, "Did you attend high school?" For those who responded "Yes," they were then asked,

"Did you experience hostility or insensitivity as a result of your gender identity or expression from other students, your teachers, or the school administrators?"

Effects of GBV on school completion. Those who reported GBV were asked, "What impact did this hostility or insensitivity have on your ability to finish high school?", with response options including, "I did NOT finish high school and the hostility or insensitivity was the main reason," "I did NOT finish high school and the hostility or insensitivity contributed to it," "I did NOT finish high school and the hostility or insensitivity was not a factor in it," and "I DID finish high school in spite of the hostility or insensitivity." (p. 470)

Mixed-methods studies, on the other hand, will describe the qualitative and quantitative study instruments in two subsequent sections.

Data Collection and Analysis

When describing the data collection and analysis of a study, some authors collapse these two sections together, whereas others prefer to keep these sections separate from one another. No matter which approach you use, make sure to clearly describe the specific steps of data collection and data analysis. We prefer to use wording such as "In the first step . . ." to achieve this goal of chronological clarity. It can be helpful to jot down the steps of your data collection and data analysis on a notepad or to bullet your steps prior to writing this section to ensure that you have the chronological order of what you did sequenced clearly for your reader. In Anneliese's qualitative study, the data collection and data analysis were in one section:

DATA ANALYSIS AND COLLECTION

Using phenomenological coding (Moustakas, 1994), we bracketed our assumptions and biases about the study before, during, and after data collection and analysis. The data collection and analysis were recursive in nature (Kline, 2008) such that earlier data collection and interpretation informed later data collection. There were four steps to the data analysis. In the first step, we conducted and transcribed Participant 1's qualitative interview. In the second step, we coded this interview and revised the interview questions according to the identified codes. The coding process began with horizontalization to identify discrete categories within the data about the phenomenon of resilience. In the third step, these codes were then used to build a codebook, and we revisited the earlier data collected and identified smaller meaning units that exemplified the meaning and essence of resilience for participants to provide a structural description for each (Creswell, 2007). In the fourth step, Participant 2 was contacted so that we could conduct the interview. This process continued through Participant 19, and each of the four steps were repeated for each participant. (Singh et al., 2014, p. 211)

In the Theron et al. (2014) mixed-methods study, the authors preferred to write these sections separately, likely because there were two types of data to describe in both data collection and data analysis:

DATA COLLECTION

Quantitative data were gathered by means of the Pathways to Resilience Youth Measure (PRYM), a composite of validated scales and sub-scales measuring participants' risks, resources, school experiences, and resilience processes. We met the participating youths in classrooms at their respective schools outside teaching time. The PRYM was administered to groups of 30 to 45 youths at a time. The PRYM was presented in English, and youths were at liberty to ask if they did not understand any words. At such times, researchers code-switched (i.e. provided a synonym in the youths' mother tongue). All questions were read aloud to the youths, who completed the measures themselves.

To generate qualitative data, we engaged with a subset of the youth participants. Those who were considered resilient by their communities— see Theron, Malindi, and Theron (2013), for a description of the criteria— participated voluntarily in "drawing and writing" activities (Mitchell, Theron, Stuart, Smith, & Campbell, 2011, p. 19). We asked youths to draw what they had experienced as nurturing of their positive adjustment and then to provide a written explanation of the resilience-process implicit in the drawings (i.e. how the experience had encouraged them to [be resilient]). For the purposes of this article, we included only drawings that reflected school experiences. (p. 256)

DATA ANALYSIS

Using the quantitative data, youths were grouped into quartiles according to their scores on personal agency within their school (overall satisfaction with their school, having a say in their schooling activities, as well as the experience of relevance and accessibility of schooling) and experiences of respect (staff demonstrated respect and sensitivity for youths and engaged in clear communication with youths). Resilience scores of those youths with the lowest and highest experiences of agency and the lowest and highest experiences of respect were compared using independent sample t-tests. Three researchers (the first author, a research assistant, and a postgraduate student) analysed the drawings and written explanations independently and inductively, using a "conventional content analysis" approach (Hsiu-Fang & Shannon, 2005, p. 1279). The process was iterative and relied on constant comparison to arrive at themes and subthemes that elucidated how respectful school environments promoted positive youth adjustment (Merriam, 2009). (p. 256)

Review the differences in how methods sections are written in your discipline by following the steps indicated in Practice Exercise 8.2 and Box 8.2.

PRACTICE EXERCISE 8.2. Method Writing Practice

Select three peer-reviewed journal articles (one qualitative, one quantitative, one mixed-methods) in your discipline. For each article, make a list of the subheadings the authors use to organize their Method section. Note the differences across the three studies, as well as the format you might like the best as a reader in terms of your understanding.

WRITING THE RESULTS SECTION

Although collecting and analyzing data can be challenging and time-consuming, writing the Results section is often like a breath of fresh air. You have already collected and analyzed your data, so really the Results section is a summary of your findings. The most pressing for you in terms of your academic writing is the decision of how to best present the data in the Results section and to be as concise as possible. In this regard, you will notice that the Results section will also differ greatly by discipline, and especially so by the type of research approach used. For instance, in qualitative studies, the Results sections are typically the longest sections of the entire paper, as the author provides thick descriptions of the findings. In quantitative studies, the Results section should be presented more briefly in terms of overall length, types of information shared, and the way the results are formatted. Quantitative results often use tables as a way

---

BOX 8.2. First-Person Narrative: Writing the Method Section

I am a qualitative and mixed-methods researcher, and I always start writing the Method section in my studies. In many ways, I have to do a brief literature review to get an understanding of the literature in an area and to submit my IRB application. However, the focus in any IRB submission is on the Method section, as the main focus of IRB review is the ethical protection of study participants. So, for myself and for my students, I encourage the writing of the Method section first in empirical academic writing. The Method section is a straightforward section with predetermined subcategories that I have to write, so this set structure helps motivate me to write. I know I just need to complete each section and move on to the next. What is my research tradition? Check. Whom do I want to sample, and what is the recruitment process and overall procedure of the study? Check. Data collection and data analysis? Check.

—Anneliese

to provide a snapshot of the data, so the reader can easily understand the findings. Unlike many qualitative studies, in which the researcher's interpretation can show up in the Results section while she is reporting the findings, quantitative studies notably do not include data interpretation in the Results section, saving these for the latter Discussion section. In mixed-methods studies, the Results section tends to hit the middle of the road in terms of length and content, as there is a reporting of both quantitative and qualitative findings. If the emphasis in the mixed-methods study is on the qualitative data, then the Results section tends to be longer, whereas a mixed-methods study focusing on the quantitative data tends to be brief, relying on tables to report the findings.

In qualitative studies, it is helpful to begin the Results section with a reminder of the study focus and with an overall snapshot of the findings. In Anneliese's qualitative study, this is how this looks in the Results section:

> Participants identified lived experiences as facilitative or as hindering gender identity development and assertion. Researchers grouped themes as supportive or threatening to participants' resilience. We worked collaboratively with participants to identify themes of supports and threats to resilience. Five themes of participants' resilience and six themes describing threats to resilience emerged. The five themes of resilience were (a) ability to self-define and theorize one's gender, (b) proactive agency and access to supportive educational systems, (c) connection to a trans-affirming community, (d) reframing of mental health challenges, and (e) navigation of relationships with family and friends. (Singh et al., 2014, p. 211)

In the Goldblum et al. (2012) quantitative study, the authors begin their Results section by also giving a snapshot of the findings, and this snapshot necessarily contains the numbers and notations of the specific statistical analysis used:

> Of the full sample of 290 respondents, those who reported GBV during school were almost four times as likely to endorse making a suicide attempt as those who had not experienced GBV ($\chi^2 = 12.80$, $p < .001$; odds ratio = 3.87; Figure 1; Table 1). This relationship held true in subgroup analyses of both trans women and trans men ($\chi^2 = 13.60$, $p < .001$ and $\chi^2 = 4.40$, $p = .036$, respectively). Trans women who had experienced victimization were more likely to have made two or more suicide attempts (45.6%) compared with 14.4% of individuals who did not experience GBV (odds ratio = 4.5). Similarly, trans men who had experienced victimization were also more likely to make two or more suicide attempts (40.8%) compared with those who had not experienced GBV (18.8%; odds ratio = 2.1). (p. 471)

See Box 8.3 for a description of how a fellow researcher approaches the writing of the Results section.

In a mixed-methods study, you will need to make decisions about not only which qualitative and quantitative results are most relevant to report,

---

BOX 8.3. Writing the Results Section

Here are my thoughts on writing a Results section. First of all, I put together the best research team I can find; this usually includes content experts, methods experts, and people that understand the end user (e.g. public health, clinical psychology, or policy). Our aim in writing results is to provide information that is accurate and useful to our readers. We understand that our work is relevant to a wide audience, many of whom may not be up-to-date in statistics, so we write our results to make sense to our reader, even if they do not understand all of the statistics used. We pay attention to having "take-home" messages. By that I mean highlighting the most relevant findings and providing the reader easy access to these findings. Finally, we have our articles read by representatives of our audience to comment on clarity, relevance, and usefulness.

—Peter Goldblum

---

but also what the best order is in which to present the findings. We recommend placing priority in terms of chronological flow on the types of data you emphasized in your mixed-methods study. For instance, in the Theron et al. (2014, p. 258) mixed-methods study, the focus was on the quantitative results, so these were reported first:

QUANTITATIVE RESULTS

Independent sample t-tests showed that youths reporting school environments supportive of personal agency ($n = 137$) scored significantly higher ($M = 129.35$; $SD = 10.57$) on the resilience scale than youths with opposite experiences ($n = 330$; $M = 108.28$; $SD = 18.72$; $t(465) = -15.379$, $p = 0.000$, η2 $= 1.99$). Likewise, youths reporting lived experiences of school staff respect ($n = 171$) recorded significantly higher ($M = 128.44$; $SD =10.65$) resilience scores than youths who had experienced disrespect ($n = 277$; $M = 108.02$; $SD = 19.08$; $t(446) = -14.518$, $p = 0.000$, η2 $=1.92$). Large effect sizes add further support to the meaningfulness of these findings. These results were consistent across all three subscales of the CYRM (see Table 1) and suggest that rights-based school environments are promotive of resilience processes.

QUALITATIVE RESULTS

We next used the qualitative data to explore what respectful teaching approaches that honoured agency of youths looked like. School environments that were respectful of youths promoted positive youth adjustment, primarily via teacher–youth interactions. In essence, these interactions encouraged youth agency, promoted future dreams of higher education and employment, and supported youths to surmount neglect and cruelty. Although we emphasize teacher actions in what follows, it is important to point out that youths collaborated with their teachers—exercising personal agency within these supportive processes. Youths reported appreciating and appropriating teachers' counsel, emulating teachers' example, and actively engaging teacher support. (pp. 258–259)

You can see that in the reporting of quantitative data, the authors use a table to refer readers to for a summary of the quantitative findings, whereas the qualitative results are reported with a more descriptive style and remind the reader about the study topic and purpose of collecting the subsequent qualitative data. The authors use concise academic writing in their reporting of findings, while also being very clear about the timing of quantitative and qualitative data collection. One thing to keep in mind is the importance of parallelism in your manuscript, and it is something that is easy to lose track of as you write. For instance, if the introduction presents concepts and hypotheses in a certain order, then the construct measures and hypothesis tests should be listed in the same order in the Method and Results sections, respectively. This attention to detail in terms of parallelism may escape writers and even editors as they revise a text, simply because they know what the text says so well, but it is the kind of detail that is noticeable and confusing to readers who may be trying to extract information from the text in an organized manner.

CRAFTING A STRONG DISCUSSION SECTION

So here is the truth. By the time you get to the empirical academic writing necessary for your Discussion section, you are tired. You have conducted an entire study, written about the literature in your area, developed concise writing for your Method and Results sections, and you are just plain exhausted. This is the main challenge of writing the Discussion section, and researcher fatigue is the main difficulty we see relating to Discussion sections that are not well organized in terms of academic writing and that are therefore difficult to follow for the reader. The good news, however, is that even though you are tired by this point (and likely burning the midnight oil to complete your writing), just as there is generally an academic writing organizing model for the previous sections of your empirical academic writing, there are some general considerations for crafting strong Discussion sections. They are as follows:

- A restatement of study purpose (in the first sentence).
- Similarities and differences from previous literature in your field.
- Implications of your study for areas of theory, research, practice, and other domains.

- Study limitations.
- Conclusion (sometimes).

The first step of any Discussion section is to remind the reader of what the study focus is, which should be a restatement of the study purpose. It is a good opportunity to remind your reader before you dive into the purpose of a Discussion section, which is to summarize how your study fits in with the overall literature in your study topic area and the overarching contribution of your study to the literature based in this area. An important way to show your contribution to the literature is to discuss how each of your findings is significant in relation to previous literature in terms of the ways your study findings align with or contradict earlier studies. Take a look at the first few sentences of the Discussion section for Anneliese's qualitative study:

> The trans youth in this study described several aspects of their lives where resilience was supported or challenged, which may assist counselors working with trans youth from a strength-based perspective. First, participants described a very individualized process of learning to affirm their gender identity outside of prescribed (or routine) navigation of identity formation. This finding is consistent with previous research by Singh et al. (2011), who found self-theorizing gender to be a key component to resilience among 21 trans adults. Participants also reported consistently using self-advocacy as a necessary strategy of resilience, wherein trans youth sought to educate other people within educational systems (Cashore & Tuason, 2009). (Singh et al., 2014, p. 215)

You can see that she reminded the reader of the purpose of the study, followed by first discussing the most salient finding and guiding the reader to learn how this finding is contextualized by earlier research to which it is similar.

We like to discuss the ways that the findings support earlier literature first, followed by any contradictions, surprises, or challenges to previous literature on your topic. A common difficulty we see in student writing is that student researchers do not discuss each of the findings—or, if they do discuss each of the findings, it is unclear how these findings relate to previous literature. The mixed-methods study by Theron et al. (2014) does a really nice job of engaging in these writing tasks in a clear and concise manner, while also guiding the reader on how to understand both the qualitative and quantitative findings:

> The quantitative and qualitative findings confirm the thesis that when schooling experiences are supportive of child rights, youth resilience is promoted. The quantitative results demonstrate a statistically significant and meaningful difference in levels of resilience processes available to youths who least experience teacher respect and opportunities for exercising personal agency and

youths who most experience these. These results point to the importance of rights-based school environments in facilitating youth resilience. The qualitative findings suggest that respect for youths is transacted in teacher promotion of youth agency and youth enactment of this, encouragement of dreams of higher education and employment and youth devotion to this, and partnerships with youths to address neglect and cruelty. Understood together, these results posit that processes of youth resilience require more than recognition of children's rights to education (see Article 28, CRC). Although access to school and learning is crucial, the results accentuate Articles 13 and 29 of the CRC. Youth participant voices emphasized that school environments promoted positive youth adjustment when they valued youths' right to freedom of expression (including being able to request support and behave agentically) and opportunities for youths to develop optimally and responsibly. (p. 260)

After discussing each of the findings as it relates to or is distinct from previous literature, it is now time for you to discuss the implications of your study. For instance, what logically follows as a result of your study that your field should know and/or can do based on your study findings? Often, study implications are discussed in consideration of the areas of theory, research, practice, and other domains. Therefore, think about what the contributions of your study might be in these domains, and if the contributions are substantial enough in one or two of these areas, this may warrant having an entire subcategory of your Discussion section to discuss these future implications. The implications sections are particularly important, as people who are interested in what the next steps are as a result of your study often go straight to reading these sections in your empirical academic writing. Essentially, your entire write-up of your study is important, and the implications section of your Discussion is an opportunity to be specific about what your field should learn as a result of your study. Hence, it is a prime chance to have a significant influence on your discipline in your study focus. Words such as *recommendations* or *future actions* are also often used as subheading titles for this section. You will notice that Goldblum et al. (2012) were very specific in titling their implications section, signaling to the reader the type of implications they would find in this section:

CLINICAL AND POLICY IMPLICATIONS

Results from this analysis are consistent with those of earlier studies, demonstrating high rates of victimization and suicide attempts and the importance of greater commitment to decreasing victimization and promoting resilience among trans youth. This commitment must be made at all levels: individual, school, family, and community. Psychologists may serve a variety of roles in promoting the welfare of gender nonconforming and transgender youth from primary providers to policy advocates (see Hendricks & Testa, in press). Every effort should be made on the part of mental and medical health professionals to identify young people with gender-related concerns and to provide sensitive and effective services. Consistent with the recommendations of Hendricks and Testa (in press) and The World Professional Association for Transgender Health (2011), counseling of trans clients should assist them in finding "safe and effective pathways to achieving lasting personal comfort with their gendered selves," as well as to "maximize their overall health, psychological well-being, and self-fulfillment" (The World Professional Association for Transgender Health, 2011, p. 1). In pursuing these aims, clinicians need to be aware that clients may have experienced prior GBV from mental or medical health professionals (Hong, Espelage, & Kral, 2011). These experiences can result in mistrust of providers among trans individuals, leading to continued reluctance to seek help. This alienation from authoritative sources of help may prolong exposure to negative GBV and exacerbate mental health sequelae, leading to a subsequent increase in suicide risk (Hong et al., 2011). (pp. 472–473)

Once you have wrapped up your study implications section or sections, then you will write your study limitations section. The goal in this section is really to help your readers understand what to avoid, consider, and do when seeking to engage in a similar study in terms of research design, study topic, or participant sampling. In plain terms, this could be titled "Stuff I Wish I Had Known" if you had a do-over for your study. A couple of key considerations for writing this section include transparency and tone. First, every study has limitations, and your reader, if he is well trained, will easily spot these, so be transparent about these. This transparency is not only ethical but also just good practice to anticipate what others might see as limitations of your study. Second, the tone you have in your writing as you discuss your limitations is important. You do not want to come off as overcriticizing or undercriticizing your study. Overcriticizing would include discussing really nit-picking items you would change that are not really limitations of the study. Undercriticizing would entail neglecting large and obvious study limitations that a scholar in your field would be able to identify. Basically, naming the limitations of your study is a good thing, and at the same time, do not sell your study short by nit-picking every flaw. See Anneliese's qualitative study:

> There are several limitations of the current study. For instance, there is an underrepresentation of trans youth of color and trans feminine individuals within the sample. Also, because the focus of the study was to identify the resilience strategies of trans youth and the researchers held significant biases that trans youth do have resilience, it is certainly likely the study does not reflect the depth of societal change that needs to occur to support trans youth resilience and minimize threats to their resilience. We used several methods of trustworthiness; however, there are always issues of response bias within the use of semistructured interviews and challenges of data interpretation that exist within a research team (e.g., group think) that might have been accounted for by an external audit of the data. (Singh et al., 2014, p. 216)

Finally, drumroll please, you come to your Conclusion section. For some of you, your discipline or the particular journal you will be submitting to may not really be fans of Conclusion sections. The easiest way to decide if you need a conclusion is to read through your entire manuscript from the potential perspective of a scholar reader in your field, and ask yourself the following questions:

- Does the manuscript end too abruptly?
- Is the Discussion a lengthy part of the manuscript?
- Is the topic of your study challenging to understand just on its own?

If the answer to any of these questions is yes, then you should likely write a Conclusion to help your reader remember the purpose of your study and the significance of your findings. This is exactly the purpose of a conclusion—to remind the reader of the overall focus and contribution of your study. Take a look at the conclusion section of Theron et al. (2014), whose study was a mixed-methods research approach in an international context:

CONCLUSION

Our study offers proof of the resilience-promoting potential of formal macro-systemic endorsement of child rights and concomitant micro-systemic enactment thereof, with particular emphasis on teacher–youth transactions that are respectful of child rights. Put differently, countries that prescribe respect for children's rights facilitate relational contexts that are promotive of child experiences of respect and healthy self-determination. Although our study was conducted in small rural communities in South Africa, transactions that endorse children as valuable, autonomous human beings can occur as readily in non-African contexts. The challenge to school psychologists is to champion school ecologies that are respectfully dedicated to promoting positive youth adjustment in child rights centred ways. (p. 262)

Use the questions in Practice Exercise 8.3 to analyze the Discussion section of articles in your discipline.

PRACTICE EXERCISE 8.3. Discussion Writing Practice

Return to your exemplar articles of qualitative, quantitative, and mixed-methods articles in your discipline. Identify the following:

- Where is the restatement of the study purpose?
- Is each of the study findings reported in the Results section discussed?
- How do the authors discuss how their study findings align with or contradict past literature?

- What study implications are identified?
- Are the study limitations comprehensive?
- Is there a conclusion section that is concise?

REFERENCES, TABLES, CHARTS, FIGURES, AND THE LIKE

Although we will not go into depth about how to address references, tables, charts, figures, and other similar aspects of empirical academic writing, we do comment on these areas briefly. There are some general considerations to follow. With references and within-text citations, you want to do a read-through to make sure there is congruence between these and that you did not leave out a reference when you used a citation within text. In terms of tables, charts, and figures, the general empirical academic writing guideline is that you are including the most significant data to report while using the most concise writing and relevant data possible. In addition, when reading through your Method and Results sections, if the information is very complex or difficult to understand in stand-alone sentences and paragraphs, then a table, chart, or figure could be helpful to use.

Overall, it is most important is to follow the academic writing style requirements of your discipline (e.g., APA, MLA, Chicago) to guide you in constructing reference lists, tables, charts, figures, and other components of your manuscript. Citation manager software can be helpful in this regard, and there are often online tutorials and exemplar articles demonstrating the use of your discipline's writing style guide that can be very helpful to consult as questions come up for you in your own writing. For instance, APA style requires that a digital object identifier (DOI) is used at the end of each reference in the reference list, and there are very specific ways to format a table to abide by APA style.

CHAPTER SUMMARY AND REMINDERS

In this chapter, we discussed the standard sections in empirical academic writing. Within each of these sections, there are not only common expected components across disciplines but also unique aspects to include based on your CoP. Revisiting published journal articles that are similar to your study can help you "see" what to make sure you include within each of the standard sections of Literature Review, Method, Results, and Discussion. See Summary Table 8.1 for awareness and action reminders.

SUMMARY TABLE 8.1. AWARENESS AND ACTION REMINDERS	
Be aware . . .	Take action . . .
Writing literature reviews for empirical academic writing can be very different from writing stand-alone literature reviews.	In empirical academic writing, develop your literature review so that it leads to your research question.
There are common subsections of the Method section within your CoP.	Read several empirical articles that use a similar research method to your study to ensure you are including all of the standard sections.
You will need to make decisions about how to report your findings in the Results section.	Depending on your research approach (e.g., qualitative, quantitative, mixed-methods), consider whether tables will help organize the presentation of your data.
When writing the Discussion section, you are guiding the reader to understand how your study aligns with or contradicts earlier research.	Clearly state in the Discussion section how the findings of your study are a contribution to your field.

CHAPTER 9

Publish, Don't Perish

Publishing your scholarly writing products takes the formula and art of academic writing to another level. Instead of receiving feedback from professors in your discipline, you move to an even larger CoP, in which you are often submitting your writing for peer review in a journal article, writing a chapter for an edited book, or engaging in other venues where your work can reach a larger audience. In this chapter, we address some basic steps for publishing your writing, return to the issue of responding to reviewer feedback on your academic writing, and describe the typical emotions, challenges, and considerations inherent in academic writing for publication. Think of this chapter as an academic writing for publication 101.

In this chapter, our **awareness focus** is on the way that publishing can feel like high-stakes work, especially because many people feel their academic and career success depends on it. Our **action focus** asks you to remind yourself that you already know a good deal about academic writing by the time you begin publishing, so remember what you already know.

GETTING READY TO START DOWN THE PUBLISHING ROAD

Within the academy, there have been generations of scholars who have heard that they must "publish or perish" to secure their careers. In other words, publishing peer-reviewed journal articles and other types of academic writing products is the name of the game. Often, this phrase also refers to number of publications, types of publications, and any number of other requirements depending on your university setting. Along the way in graduate school, you may have already begun to think about the issue of publishing in your field, as when you graduate you are expected to have a certain publication record. For others as early career professionals, you may have received more detailed information on publishing requirements for tenure and promotion. Regardless, there are some general rules you can follow when seeking to publish your work; we discuss them below.

DEVELOPING MENTOR RELATIONSHIPS AND COLLABORATIONS

Mentoring is a key factor in publishing academic writing, as many students and early career professionals struggle with what the first steps are in the process. Hopefully, you have a strong relationship with one of your professors or advisors. In this case, you can jump right in and ask your professor to mentor you in publishing, in addition to exploring various publishing opportunities with her on her own work or supporting your own publishing efforts. However, if you do not have an established mentoring relationship, all hope for publishing is not lost. Many professors welcome writing projects with students. Keep in mind that professors have typically been publishing for a long time, and there may be (believe it or not) parts of the writing process that they would rather not write. For instance, students can help with writing annotated bibliographies, literature reviews, or even revising previous work that has been written by a professor. So, whether you have a current mentor or not, ask about opportunities to work with professors and to be mentored in your academic writing toward publication. In these mentoring relationships, it is important to have discussions about authorship, work style, expectations, timelines, focus, content, and all of the other considerations of publishing academic writing. By doing so, you increase the chances of developing a strong working relationship that might even outlive the current project. Trust is a large part of these types of collaborations, and so meeting deadlines and ongoing communication are key ingredients to successful writing relationships.

In addition, academic writing collaborations can occur not only outside of work with your professor but also with professors and colleagues at other universities or with peers within your own CoP at your university. Therefore, there are truly multiple opportunities to collaborate in learning about publishing your academic writing. That being said, some CoPs frown on collaborative publishing (so, you guessed it, ask your mentor about what is best in your field). However, in our experience, especially for those new to academic publishing, collaboration is not only key to learning about the publishing experience but also an expected aspect of being a new author in your CoP. Similarly to working with your mentor, cultivating dependability and trust, as well as clear communication, provide important foundational elements of your collaboration with your peers. Talking early and often about everything from authorship order to where to publish—and even your personal preferences and coping styles (as discussed in Chapter 6)—is a great idea.

When you are seeking to collaborate with professors or peers, remember that you are learning something new and that things can go wrong. For example, there are people who we worked with early on in our publishing careers who are good people but who just were not a good match for the type of working partnerships we wanted. Even from these not-so-great experiences, however, we learned a good deal about what we need in a writing collaborator. For example, Anneliese thrives on structure and deadlines to keep her on track, and Lauren feels best in a writing partnership in which she is able to talk through ideas as she writes. Even if you are venturing into your first writing collaboration, have some up-front discussions on what is important to you and how publishing your academic writing is part of your overall career goals. These types of conversations at the outset of collaborative writing help set expectations and foster understanding of what each of you needs, and they will help you when you face challenges in the process.

THE ETHICS OF ACADEMIC WRITING

Much of the ethics of academic writing applies not only to what you individually are expected to do but also to your collaborative writing relationships. When you decide to collaborate with others, make sure to have a conversation with your coauthors right away about the order in which author names will be listed on the publication. Most disciplines address research integrity issues such as this within the code of ethics for a discipline. We have heard many stories in which people have not had these up-front conversations and are in the middle—or worse at the end—of a project and just beginning to have conversations about author order. These late conversations are avoidable, and having them early can set the stage for good, healthy writing relationships that can outlast one writing project or continue for a lifetime of research. Some students feel awkward about having these conversations, especially with their professors or mentors. We still encourage these conversations, as what you are thinking may not be what your professor or mentor is thinking, and a lot of disappointment can result when there is a misunderstanding. Also, have a conversation about what merits being an author. It can vary across disciplines, but generally it is the significant contributions to article conceptualization and organization that drive authorship; although, for some disciplines, it can be the time spent. So don't assume that if you are writing a literature review for a mentor you have authorship on that manuscript. Overall, we advise you not only to have conversations about author order early in the writing game but also to set expectations that there will be an ongoing dialogue about author order to address unexpected possibilities, because circumstances can change for authors due to workload or life emergencies.

In addition to research ethics in collaborative writing, as an individual academic writer, you are expected to produce writing that is free of plagiarism. Plagiarism includes taking someone else's words and presenting them as if they are your own. However, we think that the broader idea of borrowing or stealing someone else's ideas also fits within the definition of plagiarism. Make a good practice of also giving credit where credit is due in terms of citing those whose work you are basing your ideas on, and exercise due diligence to ensure that the ideas you are coming up with on your own are not already in existence within the literature. You are a more ethical and stronger scholar when you show that your ideas are grounded in the larger scholarship. Some students like to use plagiarism software detectors to double-check their writing, and many of these can be used online. Although we rarely run into plagiarism in graduate student writing, it does happen—especially when students are tired, close to a deadline, or feel stuck. Reach out for help in these situations. Ask for a deadline extension or talk to a peer or your mentor. Plagiarism can tank your entire academic career, so take it seriously.

KNOWING WHERE TO PUBLISH JOURNAL ARTICLES: IMPACT FACTORS AND BEYOND

In your CoP, there are going to be some general guidelines about where you should publish and the type of work you should be engaging in in terms of writing products. Talking with mentors about this topic is a great place to start. Also, noting the typical academic journals that you are reading within your topic area is important, as these are likely potential venues for your own work. Sometimes, you will be working in an area that is not only new in your field but that also draws from other CoPs outside of your discipline. In these situations, you may even consider publishing in the academic journals in those CoPs to which people in your field may not be submitting their work at all. In this latter case, again, it is a great idea to get early and ongoing feedback on publishing in these outlets from mentors within and outside of your department.

As you begin to publish, you will also likely hear phrases such as *impact factor* and *premiere journal*—or even *leading journal*—to denote the most competitive publication outlets for your work. Other terms that are common include *first-tier* journal to refer to the primary, leading journals of your CoP, whereas *second-tier, third-tier,* and so on denote publication venues that are not only not as prestigious as the first-tier ones but that also have lower rejection rates. These journals (again, ask your mentors) may be good first attempts at publishing for those early in the publication process. For others, your CoP may not value outlets that are not first-tier journals. Regardless of the tier, knowing where to publish is important. You could aim high for the first tier with your writing, then, if your writing is rejected, submit your work to a lower-tier journal. Or you could start with a lower-tier journal (or newsletter article, blog post, research brief, or other type of academic writing) and then build a publication record so that you can cite your own work in your submissions to top-tier journals.

On the other hand, impact factor may be an important consideration in your publishing. Impact factor is a fancy phrase to refer to how much potential influence your journal article will have in the field based on a fancy equation of how many times articles in the journal have received citations by other authors. The impact factor of a journal is recalculated regularly, so they can change over time; therefore, it is important to know what these impact factors are. Sometimes, your CoP may not be as concerned with a formal impact factor of a journal, as the journals in your CoP are not ranked highly in impact factor. In these situations, the influence your article may have might be assessed through readership numbers or rejection rates (e.g., percentage of articles submitted for publication in the journal that are rejected in the peer review process). Whether you call it impact factor, readership, rejection rates, or something else in your CoP, know what the important journals are for peer review, how these journals are ranked, and where those who are early in the publishing process typically submit their work in your field. Another issue to consider is whether or not to publish in journals that are primarily online. Although this concern is becoming less and less as more journals are no longer primarily published in a paper format, it may be something to think about in your CoP. One important consideration, though, is that sometimes journals in your field may not be peer reviewed or may operate on a pay-to-publish basis (e.g., as in you pay the journal to publish your work). We suggest staying away from these outlets unless there is a very good reason that your mentors suggest you publish in them. See Box 9.1 for a story of the unexpected that can happen when first seeking to publish your work.

UNDERSTANDING AUTHOR SUBMISSION GUIDELINES

Once you have identified the journals in which you want to consider publishing, then there are some simple steps. Each journal has a website on which the author submission guidelines are listed. Even if you think you are nowhere near the stage of wanting to or needing to publish, we encourage you to take a look at these author guidelines. These guidelines range from writing style to use to how to format your article and the limit on number of pages. If you are actively seeking to publish your work, follow these author submission guidelines to the letter. Many editors will reject your submission outright for not following guidelines, and even if they do not, it can be annoying to editors, who often handle large volumes of submissions,

BOX 9.1. The Wild Ride of Publishing Academic Work

I selected a manuscript-style dissertation, because I knew I wanted to publish my dissertation research eventually and did not want it to sit on a shelf getting dusty. So, in my first year as faculty, I had one manuscript ready for submission. I submitted to the journal in my field that was considered to be top tier. I was rejected. I then submitted it to another leading journal in our field, and I was rejected. I was ready to give up. Then my mentor encouraged me to look at a journal outside of my CoP. I submitted the manuscript to this interdisciplinary journal, making changes based on the feedback from the earlier two rejections. I was immediately accepted! The best news, though, was that whereas the first two leading journals had rejected my work, these journals were not ranked in terms of impact factor. However, the interdisciplinary journal had such a strong citation record that not only was it ranked in terms of impact factor but its impact factor was really high. This has been, therefore, one of my most widely cited articles, and I could have never guessed that the wild ride of rejection and revision would lead to such an unexpected surprise fit for my study in a highly ranked journal outside of my CoP.

—Anneliese

to have to focus on telling you what you did wrong, when you might have done it correctly by simply reading the guidelines. We suggest pulling two or three articles on a topic similar to yours from the journal in which you want to publish so that you can see how authors have organized their overall manuscripts, including their subheadings, tables, appendices, and overall allotment of pages so your manuscript is in the general realm of these conventions.

The author submission guidelines also give you insight into the types of sections the journal has (e.g., theory, research, opinion pieces, book reviews, teaching briefs), so these guidelines can actually help you target the type of writing you would like to submit to this journal. Many of those new to publishing will begin with a nonempirical submission, such as a book review or literature review, and there are many journal outlets for this type of submission. These guidelines will also tell you how to submit the manuscript to the editor (usually through a manuscript portal online, but some still use email submissions), as well as what documents to submit. For instance, peer review refers often to academic work that is reviewed anonymously, so that the reviewers and the authors do not know one another's names. In these cases, editors may want a submitted document with the authors' names on it, as well as one document that does not have any author identifiers on it so it can easily be passed on for peer review. Other author guidelines detail that the title page, figures, tables, and appendices must be submitted in a separate document. And it is good practice to write a cover letter describing your submission and the fit for the journal, especially if there is a specific section of the journal to which you are submitting. With online portals most frequently used by journals to accept manuscript submissions, the cover letter needs to be brief—especially if there is a character limit for your entry online. We like to include the following in the cover letter (written on university letterhead if a document can be uploaded):

- Name of editor.
- Title of submission.
- One to two sentences about the submission.
- Statement of research ethics.

See Box 9.2 for an example of a cover letter.

BOX 9.2. Writing a Cover Letter for a Journal Article Submission

Date

Dear Dr. Name-of-Editor,

I would like to submit the empirical manuscript titled "Popular Opinion Leaders Groups and the Reduction of LGBTQ-Aggression in Middle School: A Case Study Inquiry" to the *Journal for Specialists in Group Work (JSGW)*. The manuscript is a qualitative inquiry using a case study research tradition.

I have prepared this manuscript revision according to APA-style 6th ed. guidelines. I have not previously or simultaneously submitted this manuscript for consideration to this or any other journals, and I have abided by relevant ACA ethical standards on preparing manuscripts and the author guidelines listed on the *JSGW* website.

I appreciate the opportunity to undergo the review process and look forward to receiving reviewer feedback. Please do not hesitate to contact me if you have any questions or concerns about this manuscript at [email].

Sincerely,
Author Name(s)

In essence, the tiny details in preparing manuscripts for submission to a particular journal can feel like nit-picking, but taking time to attend to them before you submit will help you breeze through the submission process when you are ready to do so. And though it goes without saying, we will say this—make sure each document you submit is pristine, without grammatical errors and typos, and also follow correct writing style and formatting of your manuscript. You definitely do not want journal editors and reviewers distracted by these tiny mistakes and thus distracted from your overall work.

COMPILING AND RESPONDING TO FORMAL FEEDBACK FROM JOURNAL REVIEWERS

In Chapter 6, we discussed how to handle reviewer feedback from peers and mentors, but it is an important concern to return to when seeking to publish your writing in peer-reviewed journals. As we discussed previously, responding to feedback is important. Some new authors make the mistake of either changing the entire manuscript according to reviewer and editorial feedback or making minimal changes—or, worse, no changes at all. We encourage you to view feedback from reviewers as a conversation with them. Certainly, your work has some growing edges, and their remarks can help you strengthen your manuscript overall. However, you have also likely spent a good deal of time on your work, and therefore it is perfectly fine to disagree with them. Essentially, there may be feedback offered, but it is up to you as to whether you address the feedback or not. Below is an example from a reviewer of one of our journal articles. Notice that we listed the reviewer's comments first, and then placed our response to their comments in italics:

Comment 1: The literature on the construct of resilience should cite the original source.

- *We cited Masten (2001) as the original source of our definition of resilience.*

Comment 2: I would suggest the research question be listed in the Method section, not at the end of the literature review.

- *We made this change.*

Comment 3: Why is literature on discrimination added? This seems off-topic for your study on resilience.

- *Our study of resilience specifically examined the resilience participants had in response to discrimination experiences. Therefore, we believe the literature reviewed on discrimination is necessary to set the rationale for our study.*

You can see that there were comments the reviewer made that we believed would strengthen our study in terms of the overall argument and topic, and we said that we made a change. However, you also should note that when we disagreed with the feedback, we provided a clear reason related to our topic and rationale of why we were not going to make the change. This brings us to the topic of not-so-helpful reviews. Sometimes you will find, as you are reading the reviews, that you are wondering whether the reviewers actually read your article. We can never forget the time a reviewer critiqued our work because we had written about a feminist approach with women (the study was a feminist group intervention with women), but the reviewer questioned why we had not worked with men. Well, it seemed silly that this reviewer would have written this comment, as that might have been a great study to do—but it just was not the study we did. Yet, it would have been even sillier—and maybe even impossible, actually—to revise our manuscript based on this feedback.

It is true that most reviewers are not paid to do this work, and often the review process is an important task on their list but might not be at the top of their list. So it really is important to be able to assess whether you are receiving useful feedback or not. This brings us back to the idea of feedback being a dialogue. When we receive peer reviews, we imagine that this is not some scary person who is out to get us or give us a bad review; rather, we imagine him as a real person who is our colleague (which he is) and how we might engage with him in a conversation about each of the points of feedback. In this way, you are more likely to be open to the feedback that truly will help your manuscript and then also be able to stand your ground when the feedback does not quite fit what you know about the literature, your study, or some other aspect of your work.

Having said all of this, we do want to address the dreaded nasty review. It is possible (though usually rare) that you will receive a review that is not only not helpful but also downright disrespectful in tone. What do you do in these cases? Take a deep breath. Talk to your mentors or peers to get some perspective on the review. Then consider contacting the editor to talk about the feedback. As seasoned writers, we have not received many of these types of reviews, but it can happen, and we ultimately wish that we would never even have to address this, especially for new authors. What we want you to know is that if you should receive this type of review, get support pronto. Do not wait. Do not bury your head in the sand. Get perspective immediately, and make an action plan for moving forward.

Once you have taken time to digest your reviewer feedback, it is time to make a plan to respond. In Chapter 6, we talked about responding to each comment you receive. It is really important to clearly communicate *how* you have addressed revisions and where the reviewer can find these changes. Especially if the time between reviews is long, you can imagine that a reviewer has to reread your original work, editorial decision and feedback letter, as well as note that you made the suggested changes or provided a strong rationale for why you did not. This is a time-consuming process, so help your reviewer and editor "see" where these changes are. Sometimes journals will request a revised manuscript with a track-changes feature enabled so they can easily see the revisions. It is incumbent on you not only to point to where you made a change but also to communicate how some feedback might have led to other revisions in your manuscript. When the reviewer feedback is lengthy, we like to list the feedback and our response to each piece of feedback subsequently. However, when you have a smaller amount of feedback, you can create a response chart to quickly capture the revisions you made when it is an easy copy and paste, such as in Table 9.1.

Some people actually like to do the opposite: Create a chart for the longer feedback and a listing for shorter feedback. Think about which you might prefer; either one is fine. What is not fine is to send in your revision without helping your editors and reviewers know what you actually revised. Remember, your manuscript is one of many that they are looking at, and the more you can help them easily see how you are responding to their feedback, the better.

REMINDING YOURSELF
THAT YOU KNOW HOW TO WRITE

Throughout the revision process, it can be tempting to want to throw your hands in the air and say "enough!" That is a sign that you most likely need a break. We often see authors early in their publishing careers begin to doubt themselves as they receive feedback from their larger CoP. During these moments of doubt, the dreaded impostor syndrome can begin to set in again. We always encourage our mentees to lean into that impending doom and actively address it with the truth. The truth is that by the time you begin down the publishing road, you have done a ton of academic writing. So, you know not only a few things about writing, you actually know a lot about writing. By this point, you have read a lot of academic writing in your CoP. You have worked on honing your writing skills throughout classes and through professor feedback. You have also learned what your strengths and growing edges are as an academic writer. Now, that is a lot of work, so of course we are going to encourage you to own that you know how to write. Sure, you may still be working on growing edges—we still work on our growing edges after all of these years. It is a continual process of getting better as a writer that does not stop. So, own that you know how to write, and use this reminder to help you tackle the hard stuff, easy stuff, and annoying stuff when it comes to revising your work. See Box 9.3 to read about how Assistant Professor Natoya Haskins stays motivated to keep publishing in her academic career.

TABLE 9.1. Sample Reviewer Feedback Response Chart	
Reviewer feedback	**Author response**
Introduction: p. 5—need a citation for "homelessness" see line 39.	Added the following citation to article and to reference list: Koken, J. A., Bimbi, D. S., & Parsons, J. T. (2009). Experiences of familial acceptance-rejection among transwomen of color. *Journal of Family Psychology, 23*(6), 853–860.
P. 6—add year "Nemoto et al., 2004" (line 15)	Added "2004"
P. 6—missing an important word in the sentence: "focus on the voices of survivors and engage in a 'radical' XXXX to gain a better understanding . . ." (line 46)	Changed sentence to read: "Burstow (2003) challenged the traumatology field to focus on the voices of survivors and engage in a 'radical' understanding of trauma and trauma work by focusing on the voices of survivors and their strengths for healing."
P. 7—research question: "how do people of transgender people of color who have survived trauma describe their experiences of resilience in response to this trauma?" It seems your research question has a second important aspect that you might consider articulating here: "And what might consideration of a strengths-based approach to resilience offer clinical practitioners working with transgender people of color?" (line 8)	I appreciate this feedback greatly. Because the study is completed, I added a reference to this in the "Future Directions and Implications" section: "Finally, although the research question for this study sought to understand the essence of resilience processes for transgender people of color who have survived traumatic life events, future research should examine specific strategies practitioners may use in strengths-based approaches with this group."
P. 10—add year (Strauss & Corbin, 2008) (line 6)	Added "2008" to this.
Please clarify that you are using pseudonyms (p. 11)	Added the following sentence to the "Data Collection and Analysis": "Participants engaged in member checking to ensure accuracy of the transcripts and to select a participant pseudonym (Corbin & Strauss, 2008)."

BOX 9.3. Staying Motivated to Publish

When I first started in academia I would only write on my writing days but it felt like it would take more time to get started and reacquaint myself with the manuscript. Now I stay engaged with the pieces I am working on by writing something every day, even if it is just a few sentences. This helps me to make more progress and not feel so overwhelmed when I do have larger chunks of time to write. In addition, I work on at least two manuscripts simultaneously, which has helped me to keep my writing process going, when I want to go in another direction, I am able to shift to the other project and continue to be productive. Moreover, I am intent regarding my writing groups. I endeavor to write with coauthors who are diligent and reliable, which helps to hold me accountable and push me to complete my sections of the manuscript.

Additionally, I am starting to use writing retreats, where I meet with faculty from various disciplines who have writing projects that need to be completed and we work on our projects independently, while being in the same space to provide social and emotional support. Lastly, I set writing goals for myself weekly; these goals allow me to adjust my schedule to ensure that I have the appropriate amount of time set aside to make sure that I am able to accomplish them and continue to move the manuscript toward publication. During the last four and a half years as an Assistant Professor, through trial and error I have found these strategies to be the most useful in helping me to stay motivated and on track toward tenure.

—*Natoya Hill Haskins, PhD*

CHAPTER SUMMARY AND REMINDERS

In this chapter, we discussed how to publish, and we challenged the myth of "publish or perish." We suggested ways that you might be mentored and might collaborate on your early publishing efforts. See Summary Table 9.1 for awareness and action reminders on how to build the confidence and skills you need to enter the publishing world in your CoP.

SUMMARY TABLE 9.1. AWARENESS AND ACTION REMINDERS	
Be aware . . .	Take action . . .
When you are new to publishing your academic work, identify professors and peers who can mentor you.	Ask to collaborate on projects if your CoP values this and have explicit discussions about roles and responsibilities during writing up-front.
Learn what your CoP values in the publishing world.	Identify the important journals, impact factors, and other information about where to publish first.
Pay attention to the details when you are submitting your work for peer review.	Read and reread your work to eliminate tiny errors and ensure you are following the author submission guidelines to the letter.
Remind yourself that you know a good deal about academic writing and that your perspective is valuable in your CoP.	Develop ways of tracking your publishing progress.

Answer Key

PRACTICE EXERCISE 1.1. Identifying Text Type

TEXT 1

1. What kind of writing text is Text 1—how would I categorize it? Is it a news article, a blog, a personal e-mail, a Web page, a brochure, an abstract for a research article, a book review, part of a literature review, part of a Method section, or part of a Discussion section?

   • *Web page or brochure both seem like possible options considering the content and style of the text.*

2. Who is the likely imagined or intended audience/reader for this text?

   • *Someone who does not know what mindfulness is.*

   • *Someone who does not understand the psychological processes involved in worry and stress.*

   • *Someone who may be looking for a way to cope with worry and stress.*

3. What is the purpose of this text? Why did the author write it? What impact or effect does the author want it to have on the reader?

   • *To explain mindfulness and how it may help reduce worry and stress.*

   • *To help readers understand an unpleasant condition that they may be experiencing and provide a suggestion for how they might improve this condition.*

   • *To reassure readers that there is a solution and to provide information that helps them understand their experience.*

4. How did the author approach the topic of this text? What strategy was used to provide a basic rationale for writing about this topic?

   • *The author asked some questions about readers' feelings and proposed mindfulness as a solution to their problems (i.e., worry and stress).*

5. What type of information is included in this text? Is it all closely related to one central idea, or does the information introduce many different ideas?

    - *Simple definition of mindfulness.*
    - *Simple explanation of the positive effects mindfulness can have.*
    - *Simple explanation of why a mind focused on the past or future isn't help-ful and how to shift mind to the practice of mindfulness.*
    - *Everything is related to the idea that mindfulness is a positive coping strat-egy for worry and stress.*

6. What is the tone of this text? What is the attitude of the author toward the reader?

    - *Informative, helpful, reassuring.*

7. What is the structure or organization of ideas in this text? Does it appear to have some kind of formal structure, is it stream of consciousness, or is it something in between?

    - *Somewhat formal, but divided into two short paragraphs.*
    - *Offers an assertion (i.e., mindfulness counteracts worry and stress), explains assertion (i.e., worry and stress do not allow mind to be in present moment), offers suggestion (i.e., how to practice mindfulness).*

8. What is the style of expression used in this text? Are the ideas tightly con-nected and clearly explained in relation to each other? Are the ideas pre-sented somewhat sequentially but not necessarily explained?

    - *Friendly informative style: simple prose; use of you; use of different cases (e.g., all capital letters for emphasis), use of different font styles (e.g., **bold**), use of "conversational" punctuation like "!"; and use of repetition for emphasis (e.g., right now, right now, right now).*
    - *The organization of the ideas indicates their relationship. The writer uses direct quotations followed by answers and gives commands. The writer uses a repeating pattern for the questions and answers to emphasize the information.*

9. What kind of grammar and vocabulary are used in this text? Are the sen-tences simple or complex? Is the vocabulary sophisticated, requiring a high level of literacy, or is it more conversational?

    - *Simple conversational vocabulary.*
    - *Could be understood by someone with basic level reading skills.*

10. Based on your answers to numbers 1–9, how does this text that you are cur-rently evaluating compare to academic writing?

    - *It does not appear that the audience, purpose, content, or language of this text reflect academic intentions. The audience is clearly not academic, the tone is emotional–rational rather than just rational, there is no appeal to credible evidence, and the prose is conversational rather than sophisti-cated.*

- *This text does appear to have an argumentation purpose like an academic text, and it does use a somewhat problematizing approach to the topic, but it does not exactly emphasize or specify that mindfulness is a new or unique solution to the problem of worry and stress. The text is also structured according to logical principles of argumentation. Although the cohesion devices in this text are simple, it also demonstrates a cohesive style similar to that of an academic text.*

TEXT 2

1. What kind of writing text is Text 2—how would I categorize it? Is it a news article, a blog, a personal e-mail, a Web page, a brochure, an abstract for a research article, a book review, part of a literature review, part of a Method section, or part of a Discussion section?
    - *Seems like part of a literature review because it appears to be part of defining concepts that will be used later, which is something that is usually done in a review of literature.*
2. Who is the likely imagined or intended audience/reader for this text?
    - *Readers who require evidence to accept certain ideas as valid.*
    - *Readers whose interest in mindfulness is abstract rather than personal (i.e., how it affects "self-regulation" in generalized sense).*
3. What is the purpose of this text? Why did the author write it? What impact or effect does the author want it to have on the reader?
    - *To define mindfulness and establish that it is rational to discuss a relationship between mindfulness and self-regulation.*
    - *To persuade the reader that there is an empirical basis for discussing mindfulness (generally not considered an academic topic) and its relationship to self-regulation (an academic topic).*
4. How did the author approach the topic of this text? What strategy was used to provide a basic rationale for writing about this topic?
    - *To propose the topic (mindfulness) as a new idea ("promising approach") for the problem of self-regulation.*
5. What type of information is included in this text? Is it all closely related to one central idea, or does the information introduce many different ideas?
    - *Definition and description of mindfulness.*
    - *Definition and description of yoga and the role of mindfulness in yoga.*
    - *Assertion of mindfulness and yoga's connection to self-regulation.*
6. What is the tone of this text? What is the attitude of the author toward the reader?
    - *Informative and rational.*
    - *Readers are logical and can be persuaded through logical argumentation and the use of credible evidence.*

7. What is the structure or organization of ideas in this text? Does it appear to have some kind of formal structure, is it stream of consciousness, or is it something in between?

   • *Assertion of connection of mindfulness to self-regulation.*

   • *Definition of mindfulness.*

   • *Definition of yoga and description of its connection to mindfulness.*

   • *Assertion of yoga's connection to self-regulation and other psychological conditions.*

8. What is the style of expression used in this text? Are the ideas tightly connected and clearly explained in relation to each other? Are the ideas presented somewhat sequentially but not necessarily explained?

   • *Formal, academic.*

   • *Tightly connected through the repetition of key words (e.g., mindfulness, yoga, and self-regulation); use of nonconversational transition words (e.g., indeed); and use of passive voice to maintain focus on key words (e.g., "Yoga and other meditative techniques have been shown").*

9. What kind of grammar and vocabulary are used in this text? Are the sentences simple or complex? Is the vocabulary sophisticated, requiring a high level of literacy, or is it more conversational?

   • *Dense, complex sentences that include multiple ideas; information is added to sentences through dependent clauses and prepositional phrases.*

   • *Present and present perfect verb tenses; active and passive voice.*

   • *Formal vocabulary (e.g., utilize, contemplative, derived from, sustained, receptive).*

10. Based on your answers to numbers 1–9, how does this text that you are currently evaluating compare to academic writing?

    • *It appears to be an academic text. The audience is academic, the purpose is argumentation, the approach problematizes mindfulness in the sense that it presents it as a new solution for a problem, the tone is rational, the content is academically credible, the structure is highly organized, the style is highly cohesive, and the language is clear and sophisticated.*

PRACTICE EXERCISE 1.2. Comparing Macro-Level Patterns

TEXT 1

1. How do these headings and subheadings relate to the questions that the text seeks to answer?

   The headings of the sections indicate a progression from discussing previous research and ideas related to the research questions to describing this study and its findings to discussing interpretations of the findings. In the Findings section, it appears that the findings can be related to three different themes— the first three subsections seem to be related to the question about parents' involvement in decision making, and the fourth subsection seems like it is more related to the question about the impact of parents' socioeconomic status on decision making.

2. Do these headings and subheadings suggest that this is a particular type of text (e.g., empirical research article, monograph, etc.)? Explain.

   This text is clearly an empirical text that presents the findings of a study. There is an obvious emphasis on attending to imagined objections to the data, as evidenced by two consecutive sections that appear to address imagined questions about the data (e.g., "Ensuring Data Quality and Reflexivity" and "Limitations"). Notably, the imagined objections to the data are actually discussed before the Findings are presented. The inclusion of Implication seems to suggest that the writer provides some type of important insight gained from researching the questions.

TEXT 2

1. How do these headings and subheadings relate to the questions that the text seeks to answer?

   The titles of the sections indicate a progression from discussing the neo-liberalization of academia in general to discussing the specific effects of neo-liberalization on normal practices in academia to discussing the very specific effects that neo-liberalization has had on different types of academic bodies. The final section indicates that the writers discuss approaches to academia that would not produce the undesirable effects produced by neo-liberalization.

2. Do these headings and subheadings suggest that this is a particular type of text (e.g., empirical research article, monograph, etc.)? Explain.

   The inclusion of a section called "Research Methods" suggests that this is an empirical study. However, the absence of any sections that appear to discuss findings or results suggest that this may not be an empirical article.

3. How does the macro-structure of Text 1 compare to the macro-structure of Text 2? Are they the same type of research article? Explain.

   Similar. They both have sections that are following an obvious argument-style organization. However, Text 1 has more standard sections.

PRACTICE EXERCISE 1.3. Noticing Some Unspoken Rules of Academic Writing

1. Can you find some immediate examples of authors using personal pronouns to establish authorial voice?

   Introduction: "We tested."

   Conclusion: "Our findings."

2. Can you find some immediate examples of authors using assertive language? When do they use this type of language?

   Introduction:

   - *The language of the Introduction is mostly assertive. Most ideas are presented as "factual." Examples include: "researchers have framed";*

"willingness to seek counseling refers to"; "studies have linked"; and "Therefore, in this study, we tested." The use of assertive, factual language in the first three sentences is intended to lead the reader to see that these writers' research is simply a logical result of the facts previously mentioned.

Conclusion:

- *Does not contain assertive language.*

3. Can you find some examples of authors using suggestive language? When do they use this type of language?

Introduction:

- *Does not contain suggestive language.*

Conclusion:

- *The language of the Conclusion is mostly suggestive. There are many examples of modals and other hedging devices like contrast markers. In general, the language of the conclusion suggests that there are alternatives rather than presenting information as factual. Examples include: "Although our findings highlight . . . it might be more productive . . . rather than attempting to change . . ."; "it might be more helpful"; "it might be beneficial"; "Although it is important to acknowledge . . . distinctions . . . could be problematic"; and "Rather than categorizing . . . and automatically assuming . . . it would be beneficial to consider. . . ."*

4. Now, compare the introduction and the conclusion. Which contains the most assertive language? Which contains the most suggestive language? Why do you think this is?

- *The Introduction clearly contains the most assertive language, and the Conclusion clearly contains the most suggestive language.*

- *The purpose of the Introduction is to present a brief rationale for the research question that is based on previous research, so the intention of the Introduction is to build a factual case that supports the idea that the research question is an important and logical question. Thus the Introduction is intended to assert a case for the question.*

- *The purpose of the Conclusion is to reflect on all that has been found and/or discussed in relation to the research question. Given that history has shown that even factual answers change over time and are generally more complex and nuanced than one study can demonstrate, authors are generally careful to hedge the claims resulting from their own research.*

PRACTICE EXERCISE 2.3. Identifying and Analyzing Research Gaps

TEXT 1

1. Which sentence(s) refer to the research gap?

"Relatively little research has been done on how victims cope with the experience of having been abused sexually as a child and whether or not CSA influences a survivor's coping styles."

2. Why is it considered a research gap according to the authors?
   Insufficient research on the topic.

TEXT 2

1. Which sentence(s) refer to the research gap?
   However, according to Mutegi (2013), science education research has been unable to explain how science degree achievement is "racially determined."
2. Why is it considered a research gap according to the authors?
   Research has not produced a satisfactory answer to something that has been clearly established as a problem.

TEXT 3

1. Which sentence(s) refer to the research gap?
   The study of cities as sites of diasporic religious place making has been extended recently with scholarship on minority religious places of worship in suburban areas (for example, Dwyer, Gilbert and Shah 2012; Marquardt 2006; Waghorne 1999). These claims for space by diasporic religious minorities in exurban areas reflect new patterns of migration, transnational links and social mobility. They also reflect possibilities for the inclusion of minority religious groups in areas that were once socially, culturally and ethnically homogenous.
2. Why is it considered a research gap according to the authors?
   Recent research says something new is happening and this creates new possibilities for research.

PRACTICE EXERCISE 3.1. Noticing and Comparing Writers' Styles

For us, Text 1 is easier to understand and follow. One of the primary reasons for this is related to the length of the texts. Text 1 is shorter. Another reason is the density of the prose (i.e., the amount of information conveyed in each sentence). The sentences in Text 2 tend to introduce more new topics than the sentences in Text 1. For example, the topic of Chinese and Korean immigrant students is introduced in sentence 1, and this topic is a primary topic that is repeated in one form or another in every sentence of the paragraph.

In contrast, Text 2 introduces two general topics, research methods and literature, in sentence 1. From there, the focus shifts in the following manner: the neoliberal academy (sentence 2), neoliberal subjects (sentence 3), neoliberal geographies in the form of bodies (sentence 4), the neoliberal treatment of bodies (sentence 5), the ways that particular bodies are assigned to particular spaces (sentence 6), bodies and the neoliberal spaces of academia (sentence 7), the subject positions students are pressured to embody (sentence 8), the negative impacts that neoliberal academic spaces have on students' bodies (sentence 9), and alternatives to neoliberal processes (sentence 10). Although the ideas of each sentence of Text 2 are clearly related to one another, the paragraph is not unified around one primary topic.

Length and density of prose are part of a writer's style. In the case of these texts, we can see that we are dealing with writers' who have very different styles. Even if these writers were writing about the same topics, it's likely that they would produce texts that are distinctly different because they have different writing voices.

Sentence structure is another aspect of writers' style. In Text 1, you can see that we highlighted sections of sentence 1 and sentence 2 in light gray. These sections reflect a structural pattern on the part of the writer. The pattern in this case is the writer's repeated choice to place introductory words or phrases in non-initial positions. For example, in sentence 1, the introductory word *however* is used in a non-initial position after the subject rather than at the beginning of the sentence. This non-initial use is grammatically permissible, but it is certainly a less common choice. It is much more common for writers to place the introductory word *however* at the beginning of a sentence so that readers are immediately aware that the information that follows is in some way contradictory to the information that preceded it.

The writer of Text 1 repeats the choice of using an introductory phrase in a non-initial position in sentence 2 by placing the phrase *considered as a homogenous group* after the subject phrase (i.e., subject plus prepositional phrase). Again the placement of the information is grammatically permissible, but many writers would have chosen to use an introductory phrase like *when considered as a homogenous group* at the beginning of the sentence because they would have considered the information in the phrase background information that was a prerequisite for understanding the information that was to follow.

In addition to placing introductory words and phrases in non-initial positions, this writer also displays a preference for adding qualifying information to main clauses by using participle phrases in sentence-final positions (i.e., at the end of the sentence). In sentences 2, 3, and 6, we have highlighted this writer's use of participle phrases at the end of each sentence in dark gray. This use of sentence-final participle phrases is grammatically permissible and strategically useful because it allows a writer to pack more information into a single sentence. However, there are other ways that this writer could have chosen to add their information. For example, the writer could have chosen to use a clause or write an additional sentence instead of using sentence-final participle phrases. Therefore, it is noteworthy that this writer chose to use sentence-final participle phrases in three out of six sentences in one paragraph.

Word choice and verb voice are also aspects of style that contribute to writing voice. In Text 2, we have highlighted the introductory words *below* and *here* in sentences 1 and 6 respectively in dark gray The writers have chosen to use positional terms (i.e., terms that locate objects in physical spaces) in their written text rather than signal phrases (i.e., phrases that guide readers in the direction the writer wants them to go). The stylistic choice of positional terms is not preferred in many types of social and behavioral sciences writing because it is deemed too conversational. Instead of a positional word like *below*, some disciplines would prefer an introductory signal phrase like *in the following paragraph*. In fact, in

Text 2, the words *below* and *here* do seem somewhat out-of-place considering the complexity of the words and ideas used in the paragraph. This may indicate that the writers were trying to soften their expression somewhat, anticipating that readers might experience their writing and ideas as complex.

In Text 2, we have also highlighted the main subjects and verbs of sentences 1–6 and 8–10 in light gray. From a stylistic perspective, it is noteworthy that the writers have chosen to write 9 out of 10 sentences in active voice (i.e., the subject does the action of the verb), to use *we* as the subject in 7 out of 9 of the active voice sentences, and to use a unique main verb in those 9 sentences. Their choices contrast with writers who might have chosen to blend the use of passive and active voice to create cohesion between sentences and avoid using the same subject in consecutive sentences. To illustrate, the writers could have done the following with sentences 5–6:

[5]Taking this into account, we then illustrate the ways in which the neoliberal university interacts with particular bodies that are deemed out of place. [6]As Tim Cresswell (1996) and Linda McDowell (1999) argue, particular bodies are assigned to particular spaces vis-à-vis gendered relations, which results in certain bodies—-e.g., sexualized bodies, sick bodies, pregnant bodies, non-heterosexual bodies, etc.—being deemed "out of place."

In this new version of sentences 5–6, sentence 6 has been restructured. Rather than beginning with the active voice subject–verb combination "we follow," the sentence now begins with an introductory phrase attributing the ideas that follow to an outside source. The subject–verb combination is expressed in the passive voice and has been changed from focusing on the writers' actions to focusing on the idea of "particular bodies" which was introduced in sentence 5. This restructuring does not change the meaning of the ideas expressed, but it would represent a change in the writing voice expressed in the text.

In both Text 1 and Text 2, the writers' choices are valid variations on how academic writers might choose to express their ideas. In the particular patterns noted, the writers' stylistic choices are likely somewhat outside the norm as they have chosen less common styles of expression. Although style is only one aspect of voice, the stylistic choices of these writers is a part of the pattern of choices that forms their academic writing voices.

PRACTICE EXERCISE 4.1. Anticipating the Reader's Expectations

1. What does the author think the reader needs to know in sentence 1? What question(s) is the author attempting to answer with sentence 1?
   - *Reader needs to know what I am going to argue in this paragraph in general terms.*
   - *What is the author's general claim?*
2. What does the author think the reader needs to know in sentence 2? What question(s) is the author attempting to answer with sentence 2?
   - *Readers need to know how I am defining the terms of my claim.*
   - *What is the author's working definition of the terms involved in her claim?*

3. What does the author think the reader needs to know in sentence 3? What question(s) is the author attempting to answer with sentence 3?

   - *Readers need to know how I am defining the terms of my claim.*
   - *What is the author's working definition of the terms involved in her claim?*

4. What does the author think the reader needs to know in sentence 4? What question(s) is the author attempting to answer with sentence 4?

   - *Reader needs to know how my terms are related to the direction I am headed with my argument, and the reader needs to know that this is a valid direction.*
   - *Where is the author headed with this argument?*
   - *Is there credible evidence to support going in this direction?*

5. What does the author think the reader needs to know in sentence 5? What question(s) is the author attempting to answer with sentence 5?

   - *Reader needs to know why I am heading in this direction.*
   - *What does the author find significant about this direction?*
   - *Is there credible evidence to support what the author finds significant about this direction?*

6. What does the author think the reader needs to know in sentence 6? What question(s) is the author attempting to answer with sentence 6?

   - *Reader needs some additional clarification on my direction and the specific claim I wish to make.*
   - *How exactly does the author define her direction and her specific claim?*
   - *Is there credible evidence to support her specific definition?*

7. What does the author think the reader needs to know in sentence 7? What question(s) is the author attempting to answer with sentence 7?

   - *Reader needs to know why my claim makes sense.*
   - *What credible evidence can the author provide that her claim is reasonable?*

8. What does the author think the reader needs to know in sentence 8? What question(s) is the author attempting to answer with sentence 8?

   - *Reader needs to know some additional explanation of why my evidence makes sense.*
   - *What credible explanation can the author provide that her claim makes sense?*

PRACTICE EXERCISE 4.2. Identifying Organizational Patterns

1. Based only on sentence 1, what organizational pattern do the authors intend to follow? How do you know?

   Classification—"three distinct domains."

2. Based on the terms italicized in sentences 2, 3, and 5, are the authors following the pattern they established in sentence 1? Explain.

   Yes, they indicated that they would discuss stigma across three domains. Each italicized phrase is a domain of stigma—public stigma, stigma by close others, self-stigma.

3. Compare the italicized terms in sentences 2, 3, and 5. How do these terms compare to one another? Why did the authors present them in this order? How is their decision related to organizational patterns?

They begin with the largest domain "public stigma" and move to the mid-size domain "stigma by close others," and finally to the smallest domain "self-stigma." (The size of the domain is related to how many people are included in the domain.) It is a hierarchical organizational pattern.

PRACTICE EXERCISE 5.1. When to Hedge and Why

1. What is the purpose of the expression "consistent with" in sentence 1? Why is it considered a hedging phrase?
   - *"Consistent with" indicates some similarity with previous research. If their findings are consistent with someone else's research, this suggests validity and credibility.*
   - *"Consistent with" is a tentative interpretation. It does not make a strong claim that their findings are the same as the other findings or that their findings support or confirm the other findings.*

2. Considering the overall meaning of sentence 2, why doesn't it contain hedging?
   - *It is a factual description of the other study. It does not contain any interpretation or suggestion of interpretation.*

3. What is the purpose of the verb *parallels* in sentence 3? Why is it considered a hedging word? What is the purpose of the expression "strengthening our interpretation" in sentence 3? Why is it considered a hedging phrase?
   - *"Parallels" indicates some similarity with previous research. If their findings are parallel with someone else's research, this suggests validity and credibility.*
   - *"Parallels" is a tentative interpretation. It does not make a strong claim that their findings are the same as the other findings or that their findings support or confirm the other findings.*
   - *"Strengthening our interpretation" indicates that the authors are aware that their interpretation could be challenged.*
   - *"Strengthening our interpretation" is a cautious way of proposing an interpretation because it implies that the authors know that their interpretation may need to be strengthened due to some weaknesses of which they are aware.*

4. What is the purpose of the verb "suggest" in sentence 4? Why is it considered a hedging word?
   - *"Suggest" indicates a possibility—a possible but in no way certain connection.*
   - *"Suggest" shows some doubt and uncertainty.*

5. What is the purpose of the expression "may simply" in sentence 5? Why is it considered a hedging expression?
   - *"May simply" indicates another possibility.*
   - *"May simply" shows some doubt and uncertainty.*

6. Considering the overall meaning of sentence 6, why doesn't it contain hedging?

   - *It is part of the authors' specific claim resulting from the interpretation of the evidence that they have presented thus far. Claims may be presented without hedging as a way to persuade readers that the claim is so obviously logical that it is like a fact.*

7. What is the purpose of the adverb "apparently" in sentence 7? Why is it considered a hedging word?

   - *"Apparently" indicates that something appears to be the case, but there could be other points of view about it.*

   - *"Apparently" shows caution in making a claim.*

PRACTICE EXERCISE 5.2. Identifying Voice Shifts

1. How many voice shifts do you see in sentence 1? Remember that voice shifts can be indicated by signal phrases as well as in-text citations.

   - *Two.*

   - *One, the voice of the author interpreting recent work.*

   - *One indicated by the direct quotation + in-text citation.*

2. How many voice shifts do you see in sentence 2?

   - *It's hard to tell because it isn't exactly clear if Casteel is the voice for the entire thought or just the direct quotations, so one or two.*

   - *One, the voice of the author summarizing the positions that have been taken in the literature.*

   - *One indicated by the direct quotations and the in-text citation.*

3. How many voice shifts do you see in sentence 3?

   - *Actually, in this case, it is just the author's voice because she is discussing her own work and interpretations, but she does reference other voices that support her interpretation through her use of in-text citations.*

4. How many voice shifts do you see in sentence 4?

   - *Two.*

   - *One, the author's voice because she is still discussing her own work.*

   - *One indicated by the direct quotation and use of in-text citation.*

5. How many voice shifts do you see in sentence 5?

   - *One—it appears to be a definition attributed entirely to Casteel and the majority of it includes direct quotation.*

PRACTICE EXERCISE 5.3. Identifying and Explaining Use of Attribution

1. Read through the entire excerpt. Which sentences are likely wholly or partially the author's voice? Remember that sentences can blend voices with part of the sentence expressing the author's voice and part of the sentence expressing the voices of other researchers.

- *Wholly*
  - *1 (Uses* we *and appears to express authors' research idea.)*
  - *4 (Appears to be a conclusion that the authors are drawing from sentences 2–3.)*
  - *6 (Uses* we *and appears to express authors' research idea.)*
- *Partially*
  - *7 (Expresses what appears to be an observation made by the authors based on their knowledge of the field in the first half of the sentence, but the second half of the sentence indicates that they are expressing an idea that has been expressed by others [e.g., "have been linked"].)*
  - *8 (Uses* we *in second part of sentence and appears to express authors' research idea, but the structure of the sentence indicates that their idea is likely based on ideas of others [e.g., "given the established link . . . "].)*

2. If you found sentences that partially include the authors' voices, which part of the sentence would need some type of attribution and why?
   - *7 (The second half of the sentence would require attribution because the authors indicate that two things "have been linked," so the reader would need to know who has made this link.)*
   - *8 (The end of the first part of the sentence would require attribution because the authors mention an "established link," so the reader would need to know who established the link.)*

3. Which sentences are likely wholly the voices of other researchers? Why do you think this?
   - *2 (Uses the phrase "generally accepted," and in order to demonstrate that something is "generally accepted," the authors would likely provide attribution for the idea.)*
   - *3 (Continues with greater specificity the idea expressed in sentence 2 and indicates that there is some type of result—e.g., "due to . . . may internalize. . . ."—that follows from the idea expressed in sentence 2. An indication of a result would likely indicate the need for attribution to indicate the origin of the result.)*

4. Are there any sentences that could go either way (i.e., they could be the authors' voices or other researchers' voices)? Why is it difficult to decide the voice of these sentences?
   - *5 (Uses "for example," which could indicate the inclusion of an example from other researchers to support the authors' ideas or an example from the authors to clarify their own ideas.)*

The following is the *unmodified* version of Choi and Miller (2014, p. 341). All of the original attribution markers have been included so that you can see how and where the authors included their attribution.

[1]We also extended research in this area by accounting for AAPI individuals' espousal of European American cultural values. [2]It is generally accepted that AAPI individuals in the United States exist in a bicultural context in which they

are exposed to European American culture and their culture of origin (Kim 2007; Miller et al., 2011). [3]Due to this sustained exposure to both cultures, AAPI individuals may internalize aspects of Asian culture and European American culture (Kim, 2007; Miller, 2007). [4]Therefore, attending to espousal of both Asian cultural values and European American cultural values might provide a better approximation of AAPI's willingness to seek counseling. [5]For example, Kim (2007) hypothesized that AAPI individuals who espouse European American values (e.g., openness and change) might feel less shame about counseling and might therefore be more willing to seek it. [6]We hypothesized that European American cultural values would be associated with less perceived public stigma and stigma by close others. [7]In addition, although no prior studies have examined the relationship between European American cultural values and willingness to seek counseling, European American cultural values have been linked to more positive attitudes toward seeking professional help (Miller et al., 2011). [8]Therefore, given the established link between attitudes toward seeking professional help and willingness to seek counseling (Kim & Omizo, 2003; Liao et al., 2005; Vogel, Wade, et al., 2009), we hypothesized that European American cultural values would relate positively to willingness to seek counseling.

PRACTICE EXERCISE 5.4. Noticing Metacommentary in Academic Writing

TEXT 1

The pattern of disclosure of participants in this study corresponds to what is reported in literature, namely that family members, mothers and professionals are the most likely sources of support when disclosing (Sauzier, 1989). About half of the participants were treated for a mood disorder, which is supported by literature reporting that the long-term effects of CSA frequently include a range of symptoms such as depression (Allen, 2008; Bennett & Hughes, 2000; Finkelhor & Browne, 1986; Spies, 2006a). The most frequently reported effects of CSA are of an emotional nature. Victims of CSA experience emotions of degradation and humiliation leading to low self-esteem (Saffy, 2003). This also seems evident in the findings that just below half of the participants experienced trust as the most prominent difficulty after the abuse, about a third experienced poor intimacy and relationships, and a quarter experienced poor self-esteem. Distortions in attachment that result from sexual abuse in childhood can be toxic in all future relationships, and especially so in the areas of self-esteem, intimacy, trust and the ability to bond (Taylor & Thomas, 2003). All four traumagenic dynamics were experienced by more than half of the women and the rest experienced at least a combination

Explains how this argument is linked to other arguments.

Emphasizes the part of the other argument that provides the link.

Explains how this argument is linked to other arguments.

Clarifies how the reader should understand the authors' findings.

of two of the dynamics. <u>This illustrates indeed the</u> severe and unique psychological impact of the CSA experience as reported by the authors Finkelhor and Browne (1986).

> Emphasizes how closely connected the authors' findings are to other findings.

TEXT 2

Finally, the finding that participants accessed their spirituality as a source of resilience—which then led to increased hope about their future as transgender people of color—is <u>similar to other</u> qualitative investigations of racial/ethnic minorities who have survived traumatic life events (Singh, 2006; Stevens, 1997). Investigations of trauma and spirituality are <u>not necessarily new</u> to the trauma field. However, <u>recent literature has emphasized that</u> practitioners should explore survivors' spiritual beliefs, especially if spirituality is a social location that assists survivors in making meaning of trauma and resilience they have experienced (Brown, 2008; Hartling, 2004). Participants particularly shared that their sense of spiritual resilience was more salient than their religious coping. <u>This finding echoes Kidd and Witten's (2009) study</u> of aging transgender persons' spiritual beliefs. In this study, the authors found participants' belief systems were often nontraditional and encouraged practitioners to "be aware of the diverse and non-traditional nature of belief structures and how these mediate life course development and impact late and end of life struggles" (p. 62). Overall, <u>findings of the current study call for</u> practitioners to address how contextual factors and multiple identities intersect and influence the well-being of transgender people of color's experiences of traumatic life events (Mizock & Lewis, 2008; Nemoto et al., 2004).

> Explains how this argument is linked to other arguments.

> Clarifies that the authors are aware of previous research. Prepares readers for new perspective that authors will use.

> Clarifies that the authors' argument is based on new developments in research.

> Explains how this argument is linked to other arguments.

> Clarifies how readers should interpret the authors' argument.

PRACTICE EXERCISE 5.5. Identifying Cohesive Devices Used for Repetition

1. *"Constructive coping" (exact repetition)*
2. *It appears that* participants *is being used for* women. *(categorical noun)*
3. *"Manifested" (exact repetition)*
4. *This substitutes for the entire idea "more than half of the women manifested constructive coping, while only 42% of the participants manifested coping self-efficacy." (pronoun)*

5. *"Manifested" (exact repetition)*
6. *"These women" (exact repetition with a directional cue)*
7. *"45%" refers to women. (ellipsis)*
8. *"Self-esteem" (exact repetition)*
9. *"This" refers to the "45% [that] obtained high self-esteem scores." (pronoun)*
10. *"42%" refers to women. (ellipsis)*
11. *"Scored high" repeats "obtained high . . . scores." (variation)*
12. *"Coping self-efficacy" (exact repetition)*
13. *"These findings" refer to the idea of the high scores obtained. (categorical noun + directional cue)*
14. *"These women" (exact repetition)*
15. Participants *is being used for* women. *(exact repetition and categorical noun)*
16. *"Manifested" (exact repetition)*
17. *"Posttraumatic growth" (exact repetition)*
18. *"Which" refers to* two thirds. *(pronoun)*
19. *"Posttraumatic growth" (exact repetition)*

References

Ahuja, A., Webster, C., Gibson, N., Brewer, A., Toledo, S., & Russell, S. (2015). Bullying and suicide: The mental health crisis of LGBTQ youth and how you can help. *Journal of Gay and Lesbian Mental Health, 19*(2), 12–44.

Allen, D. (2002). *Getting things done: The art of stress-free productivity.* New York: Penguin Books.

American Journal of Education. (n.d.). Instructions for authors. Retrieved from *www.press.uchicago.edu/journals/aje/instruct.html?journal=aje.*

Berke, J. (1994). *Twenty questions for the writer: A rhetoric with readings* (6th ed.). New York: Wadsworth.

Brown, M. (2014). Gender and sexuality: II. There goes the gayborhood? *Progress in Human Geography, 38*(3), 45–65.

Bugg, L. B. (2013). Citizenship and belonging in the rural fringe: A case study of a Hindu temple in Sydney, Australia. *Antipode, 45*(5), 1148–1166.

Buzan, T. (n.d.). What is a mindmap? Retrieved from *www.tonybuzan.com/about/mind-mapping.*

Chang, M. J., Sharkness, J., Hurtado, S., & Newman, C. B. (2014). What matters in college for retaining aspiring scientists and engineers from underrepresented racial groups. *Journal of Research in Science Teaching, 51*(5), 555–580.

Choi, N.-Y., & Miller, M. J. (2014). AAPI college students' willingness to seek counseling: The role of culture, stigma, and attitudes. *Journal of Counseling Psychology, 61*(3), 340–351.

Fulwiler, T., & Young, A. (Eds.). (2000). Language connections: Writing and reading across the curriculum. Available at WAC Clearinghouse Landmark Publications in Writing Studies: *http://wac.colostate.edu/books/language_connections.* (Original work published in print, 1982, by National Council of Teachers of English, Urbana, Illinois)

Gayner, B., Esplen, M. J., DeRoche, P., Wong, J., Bishop, S., Kavanagh, L., et al. (2012). A randomized controlled trial of mindfulness-based stress reduction to manage affective symptoms and improve quality of life in gay men living with HIV. *Journal of Behavioral Medicine, 35*(3), 272–285.

Gladwell, M. (2008). *Outliers: The story of success.* New York: Little, Brown, and Company.

Glassman, J. (2010). Critical geography: II. Articulating race and radical politics. *Progress in Human Geography, 34*(4), 506–510.

Goldblum, P., Testa, R. J., Pflum, S., Hendricks, M. L., Bradford, J., & Bongar, B. (2012). The relationship between gender-based victimization and suicide attempts in transgender people. *Professional Psychology: Research and Practice, 43*(5), 468–475.

Gould, L. F., Dariotis, J. K., Mendelson, T., & Greenberg, M. T. (2012). A school-based mindfulness intervention for urban youth: Exploring moderators of intervention effects. *Journal of Community Psychology, 40*(8), 968–982.

Graff, G., & Birkenstein, C. (2014). *They say, I say: The moves that matter in persuasive writing* (3rd ed.). New York: Norton.

Grant, A. M., & Pollock, T. G. (2011). From the editors: Publishing in *AMJ*—Part 3: Setting the hook. *Academy of Management Journal, 54*(5), 873–879.

Greason, P. B., & Cashwell, C. S. (2009). Mindfulness and counseling self-efficacy: The mediating role of attention and empathy. *Counselor Education and Supervision, 49,* 2–19.

Hagen, B., Wong-Wylie, G., & Pijl-Zieber, E. (2010). Tablets or talk?: A critical review of the literature comparing antidepressants and counseling for treatment of depression. *Journal of Mental Health Counseling, 32*(2), 102–124.

Hawkins, R., Manzi, M., & Ojeda, D. (2014). Lives in the making: Power, academia and the everyday. *ACME: An International Journal for Critical Geographies, 13*(2), 328–351.

Hays, D. G., & Singh, A. A. (2012). *Qualitative inquiry in clinical and educational settings.* New York: Guilford Press.

Hinds, J. (1987). Reader versus writer responsibility: A new typology. In U. Connor & R. B. Kaplan (Eds.), *Writing across languages: Analysis of L2 text* (pp. 141–152). Reading, MA: Addison-Wesley.

Huff, A. S. (1999). *Writing for scholarly publication.* Thousand Oaks, CA: SAGE.

Hwahng, S., & Nuttbrock, L. (2014). Adolescent gender-related abuse, androphilia, and HIV risk among transfeminine people of color in New York City. *Journal of Homosexuality, 61*(5), 691–713.

Jones, S., & Rainville, K. N. (2014). Introduction: Coaches as intellectuals. *Reading and Writing Quarterly, 30,* 183–189.

Journal of Counseling Psychology. (n.d.). Submissions. Retrieved from *www.apa. org/pubs/journals/cou/?tab=4.*

Kim, E. (2014). When social class meets ethnicity: College-going experiences of Chinese and Korean immigrant students. *Review of Higher Education, 37*(3), 321–348.

Kuhlen, A. K., Galati, A., & Brennan, S. E. (2012). Gesturing integrates top-down and bottom-up information: Joint effects of speakers' expectations and addressees' feedback. *Language and Cognition, 4*(1), 17–41.

Lamott, A. (1995). *Bird by bird: Some instructions on writing and life.* New York: Anchor.

Lave, J., & Wenger, E. (1991). *Situated learning: Legitimate peripheral participation.* New York: Cambridge University Press.

Mueller, P. A., & Oppenheimer, D. M. (2014). The pen is mightier than the keyboard: Advantages of longhand over laptop note taking. *Psychological Science, 25*(6), 1159–1168.

Patel, M. N., Bhaju, J., Thompson, M. P., & Kaslow, N. J. (2012). Life stress as mediator of the childhood maltreatment–intimate partner violence link in low-income, African American women. *Journal of Family Violence, 27*, 1–10.

Rilke, R. M. (1934). *Letters to a young poet.* New York: Norton.

Singh, A. A., & McKleroy, V. S. (2011). "Just getting out of bed is a revolutionary act": The resilience of transgender people of color who have survived traumatic life events. *International Journal of Traumatology, 17*(2), 34–44.

Singh, A. A., Meng, S., & Hansen, A. (2014). "I am my own gender": Resilience strategies of trans youth. *Journal of Counseling and Development, 92*(2), 208–218.

Swales, J. M. (1990). *Genre analysis: English in academic and research settings.* New York: Cambridge University Press.

TESOL Quarterly. (n.d.). Author guidelines. Retrieved from *http://onlinelibrary. wiley.com/journal/10.1002/(ISSN)1545-7249/homepage/ForAuthors.html.*

Theron, L., Lievenberg, L., & Malindi, M. (2014). When schooling experiences are respectful of children's rights: A pathway to resilience. *School Psychology International, 35*(3), 253–265.

University of Georgia Office of Vice President for Public Service and Outreach. (2014). Faculty find common ground, collaborate after meeting on tour. Retrieved from *http://outreach.uga.edu/faculty-find-common-ground-collaborate-after-meeting-on-tour.*

Walker-Williams, H. J., van Eeden, C., & van der Merwe, K. (2012). The prevalence of coping behavior, posttraumatic growth and psychological well-being in women who experienced childhood sexual abuse. *Journal of Psychology in Africa, 22*(4), 617–626.

Wernick, L. J., Kulick, A., & Inglehart, M. H. (2014). Influences of peers, teachers, and climate on students' willingness to intervene when witnessing anti-transgender harassment. *Journal of Adolescence, 37*(4), 927–935.

Index

Note: f following a page number indicates a figure; *t* indicates a table; *b* indicates a box.

About the Authors

Anneliese A. Singh, PhD, LPC, is Associate Dean for Diversity, Equity, and Inclusion in the College of Education and Associate Professor in the Department of Counseling and Human Development Services at the University of Georgia. Her clinical, research, and advocacy interests include LGBT youth, Asian American/Pacific Islander counseling and psychology, multicultural counseling and social justice training, qualitative methodology with historically marginalized groups (e.g., people of color, LGBT individuals, immigrants), and feminist empowerment interventions with survivors of trauma. Dr. Singh is passionate about helping students and early-career professionals to develop their academic writing skills and their writing voices. She has conducted numerous seminars and workshops on academic writing at the graduate level, in addition to teaching writing courses at the doctoral level. The recipient of numerous awards for her scholarship, Dr. Singh is a prolific writer, with more than 100 peer-reviewed journal articles, book chapters, and other professional publications. Her books include *Qualitative Inquiry in Clinical and Educational Settings* (coauthored with Danica G. Hays).

Lauren Lukkarila, PhD, is Assistant Director of the Georgia Tech Language Institute, where she is also a lecturer and coordinates the curriculum of the Intensive English program, as well as many of the other academic-, professional-, and general-skills short programs. Dr. Lukkarila's research foci include feminist approaches to English as a second language (ESL) pedagogy, critical pedagogy in ESL, academic reading–writing connections, identity and academic writing, critical thinking pedagogy, and academic writing pedagogy. She has been teaching pre- and post-matriculated ESL writers how to succeed at U.S. university academic writing for over a decade. She is a frequent guest lecturer on graduate academic writing and has been honored for her curriculum innovation with international students.